D0502076

Stop Prediabetes Now

Also by Jack Challem

Syndrome X

The Inflammation Syndrome

Feed Your Genes Right

The Food-Mood Solution

Stop Prediabetes Now

The Ultimate Plan to Lose Weight and Prevent Diabetes

Jack Challem

Ron Hunninghake, M.D.

John Wiley & Sons, Inc.

Published by John Wiley & Sons, Inc., Hoboken, New Jersey
Published simultaneously in Canada

Wiley Bicentennial Logo: Richard J. Pacifico

Design and compostition by Navta Associates, Inc.

The information contained in this book is not intended to serve as a replacement for professional medical advice. Any use of the information in this book is at the reader's discretion. The author and the publisher specifically disclaim any and all liability arising directly or indirectly from the use or application of any information contained in this book. A health care professional should be consulted regarding your specific situation.

For general information about our other products and services, please contact our Customer Care Department within the United States at (800) 762-2974, outside the United States at (317) 572-3993 or fax (317) 572-4002.

Wiley also publishes its books in a variety of electronic formats. Some content that appears in print may not be available in electronic books. For more information about Wiley products, visit our web site at www.wiley.com.

Library of Congress Cataloging-in-Publication Data:

Challem, Jack.
  Stop prediabetes now : the ultimate plan to lose weight and prevent diabetes / Jack Challem, Ron Hunninghake.
      p. cm.
  Includes bibliographical references and index.
  ISBN 978-0-470-12173-3 (cloth)
  1. Prediabetic state—Prevention—Popular works. 2. Diabetes—Diet therapy—Popular works. 3. Obesity—Prevention—Popular works. 4. Weight loss. I. Hunninghake, Ronald E. II. Title.
  RC660.4.C44 2007
  616.4'620654—dc22

                                                                            2007032124

Printed in the United States of America

10 9 8 7 6 5 4 3 2 1

In memory of Hugh Riordan, M.D.,

who gave us plenty of food for thought

CONTENTS

ACKNOWLEDGMENTS

No book would be possible without the direct and background help of many other people. We would like to thank our wives, Helen and Mary Jo, for their patience, love, and acceptance of the time our work and writing take.

We would also like to thank our editor, Tom Miller, for seeing the need for this book as much as we did. We thank our agent, Jack Scovil, for his advice and mastery of the contractual details. And we thank Kimberly Monroe-Hill and Patricia Waldygo for their careful editing and appreciation of words.

There are so many people—far too many to be named—who have helped to shape our ideas about nutrition and health in general and about prediabetes, diabetes, and overweight specifically. You've given us opportunities, and you've inspired us to try to inspire others. Both of us also owe the staff, the board members, and the patients at the Center for the Improvement of Human Functioning International, in Wichita, Kansas, a huge thank-you: all the big and little things you do make everyone's life better.

NOTE TO READERS

Throughout this book we write about prediabetes and diabetes. In using these terms, we refer specifically to conditions also known as type 2, adult-onset, and noninsulin-dependent prediabetes and diabetes. We do not mean type 1 or insulin-dependent diabetes, which has different causes.

Prediabetes and diabetes are serious diseases. We ask that you work with your physician in treating these diseases and, as appropriate, share this book and the medical references at the back of the book with your doctor.

Introduction

If you're like most people, you struggle to control your weight. You may not realize that you're probably attempting to control your blood sugar as well.

In fact, your silent blood-sugar problems are a major reason why you're overweight.

This news may surprise and even shock you, but being overweight and having blood-sugar problems tend to go hand in hand. The reason is that up-and-down blood-sugar swings throughout the day increase your hunger jags, snacking, and overeating. When you eat too much and pack on the pounds, you set the stage for developing prediabetes, obesity, and full-blown diabetes.

That's just the beginning. Once you start down the path toward prediabetes and overweight, you face an increased risk of suffering from many other painful, debilitating, and life-threatening health problems. It's not a pretty picture.

The sad fact is that both prediabetes and overweight are out-of-control modern epidemics. Two-thirds of North Americans are now overweight, and almost as many people have some early signs of prediabetes. Although overweight and prediabetes don't always overlap, they do much of the time.

If you happen to be thin, don't count your blessings just yet. That's because one-fourth of thin people are also prediabetic.

What's the cause? The dual afflictions of prediabetes and overweight result from slamming your body too many times with unhealthy foods. The foods you've eaten and thought were safe have created your health problems.

Are we trying to scare you? Yes, we want to scare you into saving your life.

As bad as all this might sound, you can do plenty to change the course of your health. Prediabetes may be the prelude to developing diabetes mellitus, but you can reverse it with careful, conscientious eating habits. Even if you have been diagnosed with diabetes, you can still reduce its impact and the severity of its symptoms.

Are You Prediabetic and Don't Know It?

When doctors and health experts talk about the health problems associated with prediabetes, diabetes, and overweight, people often have trouble imagining the horrible consequences; for example, diabetes can result in blindness, nerve damage, kidney failure, and amputation. So let's take a different approach and consider how you look and feel today. Some of the early symptoms of prediabetes are so common that many people assume they're normal. These signs of prediabetes fall into four groupings.

1. Mind, Mood, and Energy Clues
Do you
- Feel tired after eating?
- Feel tired or not have much energy in general?
- Have difficulty concentrating after eating?
- Experience fuzzy thinking a lot of the time?
- Have bad moods when you don't eat on time?

2. Physical Clues
Do you
- Have love handles?

- Have a potbelly, even a small one?
- Have a forty-inch or larger waist (men)?
- Have a thirty-five-inch or larger waist (women)?
- Experience frequent heartburn or acid reflux or take meds for symptom control?
- Have trouble maintaining an erection without medication (men only)?
- Engage in little or no physical activity on most days?
- Have facial hair, plus difficulty in conceiving (women only)?
- Need to urinate frequently?
- Feel that your mouth is often dry?

3. Medical Clues

Do you

- Have elevated fasting glucose (above 90 mg/dl)?
- Have elevated fasting insulin (above 10 mcIU/ml)?
- Have high total cholesterol or LDL cholesterol?
- Have high triglyceride levels?
- Have high C-reactive protein (CRP) levels?
- Take a drug to reduce your blood-sugar levels?
- Know whether you were a low-birth-weight baby (less than six pounds)?
- Know whether you were a high-birth-weight baby (more than ten pounds)?
- Remember whether you grew up exposed to secondhand smoke?

4. Eating Clues

Do you

- Skip breakfast or have only coffee and something sweet?
- Tend to pig out while eating?
- Often feel as if you can't stop eating?
- Snack frequently, such as while watching television?
- Eat out of boredom?

- Have food cravings, especially for sweet or carb-rich foods?
- Eat to get more energy?
- Have sugary soft drinks most days?
- Eat fast foods (e.g., McDonald's) at least once a week?
- Drink beer or hard liquor (spirits) at least once a week?

If you see yourself in any of these examples, it's time to change your habits before you develop more serious health problems.

Are You in Denial about Your Weight?

Being overweight is the number-one risk factor for developing prediabetes and diabetes. You may feel smug thinking that your weight is normal, but chances are you're wrong.

Denial is a huge part of the growing problem of prediabetes and overweight. Most people think they look better than they do, assume they weigh less than they actually do, and believe that love handles or a pot-belly aren't a big deal.

In one survey, nine out of ten Americans thought that most other people were overweight, but only about half of them acknowledged that they themselves had weight problems. Another study found that a majority of people didn't think being overweight was a serious issue except for extreme obesity, such as when someone weighed more than four hundred pounds.

Denial takes other forms, too. Wearing large-size clothes, such as baggy jeans, and sweatshirts, covers up embarrassing, overweight bodies. You can buy mirrors that make you look thinner, and clothing stores routinely use these mirrors to flatter their customers. Other people squeeze their butts into small sizes just to say that they fit, although the clothes practically burst at the seams. In 2006, Hewlett-Packard introduced a digital camera with three settings to make people look thinner than they really are. "You'll trim down to a new you, instantly," said one advertisement.

People keep deceiving themselves, and they rationalize each extra helping of food, their nonstop snacking, their tight-fitting clothes, and how their bellies ache after they pig out. The more people snack and overeat, the more food they want, and the worse their blood sugar and weight become.

The Numbers Add Up to a Huge, Growing Health-Care Crisis

Maybe you need to hear a few alarming statistics to be convinced. The following numbers sent a chill down our spines, and they should be just as scary for you.

- *Overweight.* Two out of every three American adults are now overweight. One of every two overweight Americans is heavy enough (more than thirty pounds over his or her ideal weight) to be considered obese. If you're obese, your risk of developing diabetes is more than eighty times greater than that for someone of normal weight. Men fare worse than women—four out of five American men are overweight or obese. That means only one American man in five is thin today. If these trends continue, according to an article in the *Annals of Internal Medicine*, nine out of ten men and seven of every ten women will become overweight or obese.

- *Diabetes.* The percentage of Americans with diabetes has doubled since the mid-1970s and jumped by more than 30 percent during the 1990s. People then in their thirties—the first full-fledged fast-food generation—experienced a 70 percent increase in diabetes during the 1990s. Twenty-one million American adults now have full-blown diabetes, and researchers predict that the prevalence of diabetes will grow to 40 million Americans in the next twenty years.

- *Prediabetes.* The estimated number of people with prediabetes currently ranges from 40 to 100 million, depending on the study you happen to cite. One study predicted that half of all Americans would be prediabetic in just a few years. Being overweight, prediabetic, or diabetic increases your risk of dying of any cause at a younger age.

These statistics are even more disturbing when you consider that diabetes used to be a relatively rare disease, affecting mostly overweight elderly people. But as individuals become overweight at younger ages, they are more likely to develop diabetes earlier in life.

The Growth of Generation XXL

Researchers and news reports frequently describe the alarming growth of overweight, obesity, and diabetes in children. When we were kids in the 1950s and 1960s, overweight children were uncommon. Today, overweight children are quickly becoming the norm, with about one in every three American children either overweight or obese.

Being overweight or obese in childhood increases a person's risk of developing allergies, asthma, high blood pressure, heart disease, and fatty liver. In fact, fatty liver, in which fat deposits on the liver impair its function and blood-sugar regulation, has become the most common physical abnormality in children and adolescents.

Researchers have projected that one of every three people born since the year 2000 will eventually develop diabetes. Already, an estimated forty thousand American adolescents have type 2 diabetes; a generation ago this disease that was virtually unheard of in children. The latest statistics indicate that almost 3 million adolescents have prediabetes, which sharply increases their risk of developing heart disease. Because being overweight and prediabetic accelerate the aging process, these children probably won't live as long as their parents do.

What accounts for this frightening increase in prediabetes and diabetes in children and teenagers? They have grown up eating large quantities of junk foods, such as fast foods and microwave convenience foods. People who dine at fast-food restaurants two or more times a week are far more likely to gain weight and develop prediabetes, compared with those who rarely eat fast foods.

On a typical day, about one-third of U.S. children eat at fast-food restaurants. Fast-food restaurants form clusters around schools, and, unfortunately, school cafeterias and vending machines aren't much better, nutritionally. In perhaps the greatest irony of all, fast-food restaurants are common in children's hospitals and other medical centers with extensive pediatric programs. In a survey of two hundred such hospitals, fifty-nine had fast-food restaurants, such as McDonald's, located on site.

Global Problems

Americans now have the dubious honor of being the fattest people in the world; however, the citizens of most other countries are quickly catching up. Worldwide, overweight and obese people now outnumber the undernourished and starving. The World Health Organization has estimated that more than 1.7 billion adults are overweight or obese, compared with 600 million who are undernourished.

In England, 39 percent of the population tip the scales as overweight, with 21 percent obese. The numbers are rising, and projections suggest that one-third of British men will be obese by 2010. In France, regardless of what you've heard about French women not getting fat, weight problems are common. Forty-two percent of French citizens are overweight or obese, and the percent goes up to 51 percent in some parts of the country.

Since the mid-1980s, the incidence of obesity has tripled in developing nations. As people gain weight, their risk of developing prediabetes and diabetes shoots up because these conditions result from the same dietary patterns. In every case, the dramatic increase in overweight and diabetes follows the adoption of Western dietary habits, such as overeating cheap foods that are loaded with calories from sugars, sugarlike carbs, and trans fats. (Sugarlike carbohydrates mean refined carbs, usually grains, which are digested almost as quickly as sugars, leading to rapid jumps in blood-sugar and insulin levels.)

It may sound funny, but in Australia officials have recommended a full-scale effort to strengthen toilet seats to accommodate growing numbers of overweight people. Back in the United States, it's become increasingly difficult to take meaningful medical X-rays because too much body fat obscures the images. More than 120,000 U.S. citizens annually now undergo stomach stapling, gastric bypass, or other surgeries to lose weight—and, as a result, they risk developing multiple vitamin and mineral deficiencies.

The worldwide obesity epidemic drives the diabetes epidemic. In 2006, an estimated 246 million people worldwide had diabetes, a phenomenal increase from only 30 million just twenty years ago. That number is expected to climb to 420 million in less than twenty years. We believe that two to three times this many people already have prediabetes, creating the stepping-stone to a catastrophic health disaster.

If You Have Been Diagnosed

If you have already been diagnosed with prediabetes, diabetes, or obesity, you may have felt, at least at times, helpless and trapped in a body you can't do much about. You may believe that life dealt you a bad hand or may wonder why this has happened to you.

These are normal feelings, and they're similar to how people feel after being diagnosed with cancer or advanced heart disease. You may also be frustrated because you know how difficult it is to change your eating habits, to lose weight, and to get your blood sugar under control. Worse, sometimes the side effects of medications can leave you feeling even sicker.

It's not uncommon to experience a sense of defeat when you receive a serious medical diagnosis. Depressed and not knowing where to turn, many people with prediabetes or diabetes simply give up. Others react with defiance, with the attitude "No one is going to tell me how to eat!" But these responses do not realistically deal with the long-term consequences of ignoring blood-sugar problems.

In our experience, many people have been let down by the health-care system. That's because the diagnosis of prediabetes often falls through the cracks. It's all too common for people to receive a diagnosis, only to be given little, if any, meaningful nutritional advice, and the advice that is dispensed is, unfortunately, often antiquated and ignores the best research.

You Can Reverse Prediabetes

The good news is that you can reverse your health problems, improve your blood sugar, lose weight, and feel more energized than you have in years.

The program we describe in *Stop Prediabetes Now* focuses on eating habits, nutritional supplements, and light physical activity. We clearly explain exactly what to do to straighten out your eating habits. Taking this approach is two to three times more effective than any medical treatment in preventing the progression of prediabetes and diabetes. The research and the experience of other doctors clearly back us up.

We're not going to ask you to "go on a diet." That's because most people soon go off their diets and return to the habits that made them sick in the first place. Nor will we promise that you'll look like a runway model or a hunk with six-pack abs. That's simply unrealistic.

Instead, we ask you to work with us to develop a new lifelong style of eating for better health. When you adopt new and better eating habits, you will likely see benefits in how you feel within a day or two, usually with impressive changes by the end of the first week, followed by many additional improvements after weeks and months. Instead of complaining about side effects, people happily tell us about side benefits—unexpected improvements in their nagging health problems.

You may think that it will be hard to make the dietary changes you need to restore your health. After all, you really love to eat, and you love the foods that are bad for you. Yet continuing to eat the way you have been guarantees that your prediabetes will turn into diabetes, most likely within the next several years. Likewise, if you improve your eating habits for a while but then return to the way you used to eat, you will jump back on the fast track toward diabetes.

There is simply no better treatment for prediabetes and being overweight than cultivating better eating habits and making other lifestyle changes. Consider just two studies that clearly show this to be true. In 2006, researchers reported in the *American Journal of Clinical Nutrition* that a combination of improved eating habits and light physical activity eliminated symptoms of prediabetes in two-thirds of the study's participants. In just six months, the participants lost significant amounts of weight, and their blood sugar, blood fats, and blood pressure decreased. Another study, published in the *New England Journal of Medicine*, found that eating healthier foods and going for regular walks were twice as effective as medications in preventing diabetes.

We believe you'll find our recommendations easier to follow than you might imagine, with meal plans consisting of tasty and satisfying foods. It may surprise you to learn that we're speaking from personal experience. That's right—we, too, had signs of prediabetes until we changed our eating habits.

JACK'S STORY

Ten years ago, I had a potbelly that seemed to grow another inch with each passing year. I felt tired all the time. And then a simple blood test told me what I didn't want to hear: I was prediabetic.

Today, I'm trim, my blood-sugar level is normal, and I feel absolutely great. Most people assume that I'm ten years younger than I actually am. I turned my life around without taking drugs or following fad diets. Granted, I didn't accomplish all this overnight, but if I can make these changes, so can you.

For years I had taken various vitamin supplements, but I paid little attention to what I was eating. By the mid-1990s, I was in denial of having a cluster of prediabetic symptoms (insulin resistance, belly fat, increasing blood pressure, and elevated cholesterol and triglycerides). My intraocular eye pressure, a risk factor for glaucoma, was also elevated at 21 and 22 mgHg.

In 1997, I went to the Center for the Improvement of Human Functioning International, where Hugh Riordan, M.D., oversaw the most comprehensive medical and nutritional workup I had ever experienced. At the time, I had a thirty-eight-inch waist and, at 170 pounds, was about twenty pounds overweight, with a body mass index of 27.

My fasting blood sugar was 111 mg/dl, which is prediabetic, and my cholesterol and triglycerides were also high. My body's levels of chromium, zinc, and magnesium, the minerals involved in managing blood sugar, were low. A dietary analysis found that I was eating too many refined, sugarlike carbohydrates, including pasta and fruit juices.

I knew what all of the test numbers meant. I was in my mid-forties and a disaster waiting to happen. Worse, I was embarrassed. After all, I earn my living as a health writer. If I couldn't keep myself healthy, what right did I have to give others advice?

When I got home, I increased my intake of alpha-lipoic acid, an antioxidant known for improving glucose tolerance. But it took me two years to figure out what to do about my eating habits. In 1999, I began writing a book titled *Syndrome X*, which was essentially about prediabetes, yet I was still in denial about having the early stages of Syndrome X, a form of prediabetes.

At that time, my personal life and relationships were undergoing big changes, and, for some inexplicable reason, I lost my taste for pasta, which had been one of my favorite foods. I started to eat more salads and baked chicken. Over the next three months, I lost twenty pounds without trying, and my body mass index decreased to 23.5, which is within the normal range. When I had my blood sugar checked a few months later, I discovered that it had decreased 24 points to 87 mg/dl. It was a significant change—without much effort.

Over the next couple of years, I made a point of cutting back even more on refined sugarlike carbs, such as pasta, pizza, bread, tortillas, pitas, cereals, muffins, and bagels. My eating habits emphasized fresh fish, chicken, a lot of vegetables, and small amounts of brown rice or yams. Follow-up tests at the Center for the Improvement of Human Functioning International indicated modest improvements in my mineral levels, but my cholesterol and triglycerides were still high, at 265 mg/dl and 174, respectively.

In 2003, blood tests showed significant improvements. My fasting blood sugar was down to 84 mg/dl, and my HbA_{1c} (a snapshot of average blood-sugar levels over a six-week period) was a respectable 5.2 percent. By this time, I had become interested in fasting insulin, and mine was good at 8.4 mcIU/ml. (I suspect that my insulin levels had previously been much higher.) My intraocular eye pressure had decreased and was now 15 mmHg in both eyes—normal!

In 2003, I began bicycling three mornings a week. Up to that point, I had been pretty much a couch potato except for an occasional long walk or hike. Another battery of tests in 2005 indicated still more improvements, mostly because of increased physical activity.

My fasting blood sugar was now down a couple of more points to 82 mg/dl—perfect normal. My HbA_{1c} was stable at 5.2 percent, and my fasting insulin had decreased to 4.9 mcIU/ml, which was superb. In addition, my cholesterol was down to 203 mg/dl and my triglycerides had declined to 78 mg/dl. Dr. Ron (as patients refer to Dr. Hunninghake) and I were talking about my medical chart and the many improvements since my first visit in 1997. "Jack, you have absolutely no signs of insulin resistance or prediabetes," he said. "You're in incredibly good health."

In my latest round of tests, in April 2007, my numbers continued to improve. My blood sugar and insulin remained low, and my HbA_{1c} had finally decreased from 5.2 percent to 4.9 percent (the equivalent of a 77 mg/dl blood-sugar level). My iron levels were a quarter of what they were ten years before; this is important because high iron levels are a risk factor for diabetes and heart disease. My cholesterol level was down to 185 mg/dl. A separate eye exam found that my intraocular pressure was just 10 in both eyes. All of these improvements showed my health to be normal, although I must remain vigilant because of my risk of redeveloping prediabetes.

DR. RON'S STORY

Ten years ago, I met Jack for the first time when he visited the Center for the Improvement of Human Functioning International, the nonprofit nutritional medicine center where I work in Wichita, Kansas. As one of the center's physicians, I often focused more on the health of my patients than on my own. After lunch, I would usually "brown out"—I had difficulty concentrating and wanted to take a nap. I did my best to hide my tiredness from patients.

Jack and I began a remarkable collaboration as friends, as patient and physician, and now as coauthors. His insights into blood-sugar problems intrigued me and prompted me to further explore my own risk for prediabetes and that of my patients. I started to check my own blood-sugar and insulin levels and paid close attention to how I felt after eating.

In the process, I realized that I was carbohydrate sensitive— that is, my body tended to overreact when I ate too many carbs or sugars. I discovered that I felt much better eating healthy proteins and high-fiber vegetables, which work together to stabilize blood-sugar levels. Following this approach, I now remain mentally sharp and physically energized after lunch.

Why We Wrote This Book

There's no shortage of weight-loss books—one sign of the enormity of the problem and the lack of genuine solutions. Likewise, there are also many books on dealing with prediabetes and diabetes.

We've looked at these books and, quite frankly, we found most of them lacking. Some of the books did a great job of explaining the problem but didn't offer any solutions. Others recommended diets that were high in refined carbohydrates (breads, pastas, muffins, bagels), which make both prediabetes and weight problems worse, not better.

Some authors gave vague advice and not enough practical information. Others wrote in such excruciating detail that their plans were nearly impossible to follow. For example, just when people got the hang of counting calories or carbs, a slew of new books asked them to start tracking the glycemic index of foods. Most people don't need more numbers to calculate and another hoop to jump through!

How *Stop Prediabetes Now* Is Different

When we strip away all the research and studies, the clinical experiences and case histories, we are always left with one fundamental, inescapable fact: what we eat provides the biochemical building blocks for our entire bodies. Eating mostly nutritious foods creates a strong foundation and frame, leading to good health and resistance to disease. Eating poor-quality junk foods, however, is comparable to building a house with a shoddy foundation and frame. The key to recovering from prediabetes is using better building materials for the body—swapping healthy foods for the unhealthy ones.

In the first chapter of *Stop Prediabetes Now*, we explain how the intertwined problems of overweight and prediabetes have gotten out of hand. There are quizzes to help you assess your risk of developing pre-diabetes or weight problems and a description of the most important medical tests for detecting prediabetes.

In the second and third chapters, we write about food addictions—why people just can't stop eating, and we tell you why some types of calories are worse than others in causing weight gain. We explain how food companies tempt people with practically irresistible foods and then accept no responsibility for contributing to prediabetes and overweight. Certain types of foods actually promote hunger, leading to increased food consumption, obesity, and prediabetes.

In the rest of the book, we coach you on how to prevent and reverse prediabetes and lose weight. To jump-start our recommendations, we list some of the foods that actually curb appetite. When you eat less, both your weight and your blood sugar will improve. We advise you on how to be a smarter shopper—what foods to avoid and which ones you can safely eat. We take a similar approach to ordering in restaurants so that you aren't sabotaged when eating out. We also explain some of the basics of preparing healthy, simple, and quick meals at home.

We recommend scientifically supported nutritional supplements that can also help to reduce your appetite and improve your blood-sugar and insulin levels. We describe ways you can increase your physical activity without having to suffer, feel embarrassed, or become a "gym rat." We provide tips to reduce stress, improve your sleep, and mellow out mood problems caused by blood-sugar swings.

Make a Choice for Health

Recently, we had dinner with a psychologist who happened to be having a particularly difficult day. She had begun her morning with coffee and cereal, had skipped lunch, and was crashing with low blood sugar and fatigue by the time we met. Before the food arrived, she drank a beer and munched on corn chips. Inevitably, we started to talk about nutrition, and Jack commented on how fast-food restaurants serve nutritionally poor-quality foods.

Barbara snapped at him and said that people have to take responsibility for their actions and what they eat, completely missing the irony of her own situation. Jack pointed out that nutrition is not taught in most schools, and many people don't understand the nutritional differences between a fast-food lunch and a healthier meal. Only when people realize that some foods are healthier than others do they know that they have choices.

We're all blessed with the ability to make choices. By reading this book, you are choosing to have healthy blood-sugar levels and weight. We're proud of you for making that decision.

What We Ask of You

People often go to doctors or other health-care providers much the same way that they go to car mechanics. They bring in their bodies and say the equivalent of "It's not running right. Fix it." They absolve themselves of any personal responsibility for what's wrong and then go home and only half-heartedly follow the doctor's advice. We call this "poor compliance."

At the Center for the Improvement of Human Functioning International, Dr. Ron encourages patients to become "co-learners" who get actively involved in identifying the causes of and the solutions to their health problems. They become passionate about regaining and maintaining good health. Over and over again, Dr. Ron and other health-care professionals at the center have seen the dramatic shift that occurs when a patient becomes a co-learner—a whole new world of empowerment opens up!

As people gain an understanding of how food affects their health, they become more motivated to stay on a healthy eating plan. This understanding can be general, such as knowing that sugar and sugarlike carbs make a person sick, or it can be a little more detailed in terms of nutritional biochemistry.

We would like you to become a co-learner with us as well. We will offer plenty of advice, but, in the end, you alone will make the final decision to control the course of your health.

Like anything else that you study for the first time, there's a learning curve. As you adopt the new habits detailed in *Stop Prediabetes Now*, they will become second nature. Your health will improve and you'll have a wonderful sense of accomplishment.

PART ONE

Prediabetes and Overweight

Two Sides of the Same Disease

1

The Prediabetes Problem

If you have prediabetes or are overweight, you have an opportunity to turn your life around and improve your health. This opportunity won't last long, and the longer you wait, the more difficult it will be to regain your health. If you have already been diagnosed with the more serious diabetes mellitus and obesity, you can still take big steps to reduce your symptoms and the risk of developing serious complications.

The alternative is to continue with your present lifestyle and get sicker. Our sincere hope is that you choose to work with us and follow our advice to get better.

In this chapter we cover the basics about prediabetes and overweight but with an approach and a perspective that may be new to you.

What Do We Mean by Diabetes and Prediabetes?

Diabetes is characterized by two factors: abnormally high blood-sugar (glucose) levels, either before breakfast or after eating, and abnormally high levels of insulin (a hormone that normally helps your body to use blood sugar). In prediabetes, blood-sugar or insulin levels, or both, have begun to creep up.

Normally, blood sugar serves as one of your body's main fuels. Without it, you wouldn't have the energy to walk or think. But when blood-sugar levels are too high or too low, you cannot function at your best.

Insulin is also essential in normal health, but high levels lead to many health problems. In fact, elevated insulin usually precedes increases in blood sugar and can serve as a reliable early warning of diabetes risk. We'll explain more about blood sugar and insulin later in this chapter.

The Journey from Prediabetes to Diabetes

It helps to visualize diabetes as a continuum. Early in the disease process, your blood sugar may rise a little too much after you eat a lot of sugars or carbs, making you feel drowsy. At this stage you don't have any formal disease and blood-sugar tests would likely look normal, but we would describe you as being prediabetic. Your body is offering clues, if you pay attention, that you don't handle sugar and carbs very well.

If you ignore these clues, continue to eat whatever you want, and neglect your health in other ways, your sugar and carbohydrate intolerance will get worse. After a few years, your fasting blood sugar will creep up until you get a formal diagnosis of prediabetes. If you ignore this diagnosis, your symptoms will turn into type 2 diabetes, a far more serious disease. If you fail to properly treat type 2 diabetes, it may evolve into a truly horrible combination of type 2 and insulin-dependent type 1 diabetes.

This progression is inevitable if you continue to eat what you have been eating. The sooner you recognize what is happening and take steps to improve your health, the sooner you can take control of your health and your life.

Doctors use a variety of terms to describe prediabetes, with the differences usually reflecting the way they diagnose it. Sometimes this name game becomes confusing for patients. All of the following terms refer to prediabetes.

- Impaired fasting glucose
- Impaired glucose tolerance

> **QUICK TIP**
>
> **What's the Difference between Blood Sugar and Glucose?**
>
> There's no difference at all, and both terms are used interchangeably. Glucose is a type of sugar that functions as blood sugar.

> ## QUICK TIP
>
> ### Understanding Glucose Tolerance and Intolerance
>
> People often talk about glucose tolerance and glucose intolerance, and it's important to understand what these terms mean. If you have been called glucose tolerant, your body can deal with large amounts of sugars and carbohydrates, at least for now. (That could change in the next few years.) If you have glucose intolerance or have been called glucose intolerant, you are actually prediabetic. The terms *glucose tolerant* and *intolerant* are a little misleading. The terms *sugar intolerant* and *carbohydrate intolerant*, or *sugar sensitive* and *carbohydrate sensitive*, may be more accurate.

- Hyperinsulinemia
- Insulin resistance
- Hypoglycemia
- Metabolic syndrome
- Syndrome X
- Metabolic Syndrome X
- Insulin resistance syndrome

If your doctor has used any of these terms to describe your health, you have prediabetes.

What Do We Mean by Overweight and Obesity?

Many people aren't always clear about what doctors and health experts mean when they talk about overweight and obesity. Part of the problem is that people frequently have distorted views of their own weight, so they think they weigh less than they do. For example, we've seen plenty of men who are physically strong but also terribly overweight.

Doctors use a variety of height-weight charts and body-fat or body mass indicators to determine whether patients are overweight. While none of these methods is perfectly accurate, they do help people assess their weight.

If you're above your ideal weight, odds are that you're overweight. If you have love handles, you're not cute—you're overweight. As a general rule, if you're roughly thirty or more pounds above your ideal weight, you're obese. If you're a hundred or more pounds over your ideal weight, you're morbidly obese.

How to Measure Your Body Mass Index

Using the body mass index (BMI) is one of the most common ways of calculating whether a person's weight is normal or not. You need to know

Determining Your Body Mass Index

BMI	19	20	21	22	23	24	25	26	27	28	29	30	31	32	33	34	35
Height in inches							Body weight in pounds										
58	91	96	100	105	110	115	119	124	129	134	138	143	148	153	158	162	167
59	94	99	104	109	114	119	124	128	133	138	143	148	153	158	163	168	173
60	97	102	107	112	118	123	128	133	138	143	148	153	158	163	168	174	179
61	100	106	111	116	122	127	132	137	143	148	153	158	164	169	174	180	185
62	104	109	115	120	126	131	136	142	147	153	158	164	169	175	180	186	191
63	107	113	118	124	130	135	141	146	152	158	163	169	175	180	186	191	197
64	110	116	122	128	134	140	145	151	157	163	169	174	180	186	192	197	204
65	114	120	126	132	138	144	150	156	162	168	174	180	186	192	198	204	210
66	118	124	130	136	142	148	155	161	167	173	179	186	192	198	204	210	216
67	121	127	134	140	146	153	159	166	172	178	185	191	198	204	211	217	223
68	125	131	138	144	151	158	164	171	177	184	190	197	203	210	216	223	230
69	128	135	142	149	155	162	169	176	182	189	196	203	209	216	223	230	236
70	132	139	146	153	160	167	174	181	188	195	202	209	216	222	229	236	243
71	136	143	150	157	165	172	179	186	193	200	208	215	222	229	236	243	250
72	140	147	154	162	169	177	184	191	199	206	213	221	228	235	242	250	258
73	144	151	159	166	174	182	189	197	204	212	219	227	235	242	250	257	265
74	148	155	163	171	179	186	194	202	210	218	225	233	241	249	256	264	272
75	152	160	168	176	184	192	200	208	216	224	232	240	248	256	264	272	279
76	156	164	172	180	189	197	205	213	221	230	238	246	254	263	271	279	287

The body mass index (BMI) is a fairly accurate way of determining whether you are overweight. Use your finger to find your height and then follow the line to the right to find your weight. Next, move your finger up to the top line (BMI). If your BMI is higher than 25, you are overweight. If your BMI is higher than 30, you are obese.

only your weight (using an accurate bathroom scale) and your height. BMI estimates are generally accurate, except for body builders or serious athletes, in which case muscle, not fat, accounts for the excess weight.

Your Body Proportions and Diabetes Risk

Although the BMI gives you a general idea of whether your weight is normal, we've found that body proportions often serve as a better guide to determining whether you might be prediabetic.

To explain, some people tend to gain weight in the buttocks, while others gain it around the belly. Belly fat is the better indicator of prediabetes and diabetes risk.

People with big rear ends tend to have a pear or pyramid shape, whereas those with a big belly have an apple or diamond shape. The diamond-apple shape points to prediabetes, diabetes, and what is sometimes called metabolic syndrome and Syndrome X. Belly fat results from two particular types of fat deposits. Subcutaneous fat is stored under the skin of the belly, and visceral fat is intertwined around organs in the midsection. Both subcutaneous and visceral fat secrete inflammation-causing substances that further harm the body.

Measuring Your Body Proportions and Belly Fat

How do you measure your belly fat? The simplest method is to stand naked in front of a mirror without sucking in your gut. If your belly sticks out from your chest (not counting your breasts, if you're a woman), you have too much belly fat.

Another way is to measure your waist, but don't use your belt size. Men tend to wear their belts below their waists, leading them to think they're thinner than they really are.

To accurately measure your waist, use a cloth tape measure. Place one end of the tape measure on top of your belly button, wrap it around your back, and match up the other end at your belly button. Don't suck in your belly as you take this measurement. If you're a man with a waist larger than forty inches or a woman with a waist larger than thirty-five inches, you have a high risk of developing prediabetes and diabetes, as well as heart disease.

For a more precise calculation, you can measure your waist-hip ratio. The bigger your waist, relative to your hips, the greater your risk of developing prediabetes, diabetes, and heart disease. Follow the previous instructions to measure your waist. Next, measure your hip circumference toward the top of your buttocks.

Now use a calculator to divide your waist measurement by your hip measurement. For example, if your waist is fifty-four inches and your hips are forty inches, your waist-hip ratio is 1.35. Here is what the different ratios mean:

- If your ratio is 0.95 (men) or 0.80 (women) or less, you have a low risk of developing prediabetes and diabetes and are not overweight.
- If your ratio is 0.96 to 1.0 (men) or 0.81 to 0.85 (women), you have a moderate risk.
- If your ratio is 1.1 (men) or 0.86 (women) or higher, you have a high risk.

Are You Prediabetic or Overweight? Take the Quiz

We would like you to take a few minutes to answer the questions on the following quizzes, which assess your risk of being prediabetic or overweight. The first two quizzes are for women, and the second two are for men. (Some questions are identical, but others differ.) Be honest in your answers. No one except you has to see them.

The Prediabetes Quiz for Women

My doctor has told me that either my blood sugar (glucose)　　Y/N
　or my insulin is high.

I've been diagnosed with either carpal tunnel syndrome　　Y/N
　or Bell's palsy.

I think my belly is too big.　　Y/N

My waist is more than thirty-five inches (eighty-nine cm)   Y/N
    around.

I often skip breakfast, except for coffee.   Y/N

I often skip breakfast or just eat something starchy, like   Y/N
    a bagel or a muffin.

I often skip breakfast to lose weight.   Y/N

I get tired and sleepy after eating, especially after lunch.   Y/N

I often feel like taking a nap during the day or the   Y/N
    early evening.

I have trouble falling asleep at night.   Y/N

I have trouble getting up in the morning and must have   Y/N
    some coffee or a soft drink to fully wake up.

I often have food cravings, especially for something sweet,   Y/N
    and have trouble resisting these foods.

I snack a lot late at night.   Y/N

I often crave starchy foods, such as pasta, pizza, or bread.   Y/N

I have to add sugar to my coffee or tea, or it tastes too bitter. Y/N

I drink one or two cans or bottles of some type of *non*diet   Y/N
    soft drink each day.

I usually have some sort of dessert or other sweet food   Y/N
    at least once a day.

I often feel stressed out.   Y/N

I seem to have a lot less energy than other people my age.   Y/N

I'm usually too tired to exercise, or I don't have enough time.   Y/N

I am usually very thirsty.   Y/N

I urinate a lot.   Y/N

I have mood swings one or more times each week, going   Y/N
    from calm to irritable or from upbeat to depressed.

I've been told that my blood pressure, cholesterol, or   Y/N
    triglycerides are higher than they should be (without
    taking medications).

Between the ages of forty-five and fifty-five, I was diagnosed   Y/N
   with low thyroid and also went through perimenopause.

A brother, a sister, or a parent was diagnosed with diabetes.   Y/N

Interpretation: If you answered "yes" to any of these questions, there's a good chance that you have, or are at risk of developing, prediabetes. If you answered "yes" to more than five of the questions, you have a very high risk of being prediabetic.

The Overweight and Obesity Quiz for Women

I know that I am overweight.   Y/N

I was told by my doctor that I should lose some weight.   Y/N

I carry my extra weight around my belly.   Y/N

I weigh more than I would like to.   Y/N

I've found that most diets don't work for very long.   Y/N

I wear larger clothing sizes than I'd like to.   Y/N

I think a lot of other people are way too thin.   Y/N

I think it's normal to gain weight as we get older.   Y/N

I have trouble getting in and out of my car.   Y/N

I like big cars because I have more room in them.   Y/N

I feel as though airline seats are not wide enough for me.   Y/N

I spend a lot of time thinking about what I'm going to eat   Y/N
   later.

I often continue to eat even after I feel full—it's hard to   Y/N
   stop eating.

I sometimes "pig out" at meals.   Y/N

I have regular food cravings, or I sometimes binge on   Y/N
   individual foods.

If I have to walk any kind of distance, I feel my heart   Y/N
   beating and feel out of breath.

Interpretation: If you answered "yes" to any of the first six questions, you have a weight problem and you know it. If you answered "no" to the first six questions but did answer "yes" to two or more of the remaining questions, there's a good chance that you're overweight but may be in denial of it.

The Prediabetes Quiz for Men

My doctor has told me that either my blood sugar (glucose) or my insulin is high.	Y/N
I've been diagnosed with either carpal tunnel syndrome or Bell's palsy.	Y/N
I'm heavier than I should be around my belly.	Y/N
My waist is more than forty inches (101 cm) around.	Y/N
I often skip breakfast, except for coffee.	Y/N
I often skip breakfast or just eat something starchy, like a bagel or a muffin.	Y/N
I get tired and sleepy after eating, especially after lunch.	Y/N
I often need to take a nap during the day or the early evening.	Y/N
I have trouble falling asleep at night.	Y/N
I have trouble getting up in the morning and must have some coffee or a soft drink to fully wake up.	Y/N
I often have food cravings, especially for something sweet, and have trouble resisting these foods.	Y/N
I snack a lot late at night.	Y/N
I often crave starchy foods, such as pasta, pizza, or bread.	Y/N
I have to add sugar to my coffee or tea, or it tastes too bitter.	Y/N
I drink one or two cans or bottles of some type of *non*diet soft drink each day.	Y/N
I usually have some sort of dessert or other sweet food at least once a day.	Y/N
I often feel stressed out.	Y/N
I seem to have a lot less energy than other people my age.	Y/N
I'm usually too tired to exercise, or I don't have enough time.	Y/N

My interest in sex is not as great as it used to be, or I have   Y/N
  trouble getting and maintaining an erection unless I
  take medication.

I have mood swings one or more times each week, going   Y/N
  from calm to irritable or from upbeat to depressed.

I get angry a lot at family members, coworkers, and   Y/N
  other drivers.

I am usually very thirsty.   Y/N

I urinate a lot.   Y/N

I've been told that my blood pressure, cholesterol, or   Y/N
  triglycerides are higher than they should be (without
  taking medications).

A brother, a sister, or a parent was diagnosed with diabetes.   Y/N

Interpretation: If you answered "yes" to any of these questions, there's a good chance that you have, or are at risk of developing, prediabetes. If you answered "yes" to more than five of the questions, you have a very high risk of having prediabetes.

The Overweight and Obesity Quiz for Men

I know that I am overweight.   Y/N

I was told by my doctor that I should lose some weight.   Y/N

I have a little paunch, but it's not all that bad.   Y/N

People have told me that my love handles are cute.   Y/N

I have to admit that I've got a pretty good size beer belly.   Y/N

I weigh more than I did in my early twenties.   Y/N

I think it's normal to gain weight as we get older.   Y/N

I wear a larger belt size than I did ten years ago.   Y/N

I wear larger clothes (e.g., shirt size or pants waist size) than   Y/N
  I did ten years ago.

I have trouble finding shirts that fit or comfortably closing   Y/N
  the top button on business shirts.

I think thin guys tend to look weak or effeminate.   Y/N

I prefer driving large cars, such as an SUV or a full-size pickup truck because I have more room in them.   Y/N

I have trouble getting in and out of my car.   Y/N

I feel as though airline seats are not wide enough for me.   Y/N

If I have to walk any kind of distance, I feel my heart beating and feel out of breath.   Y/N

I often continue to eat even after I feel full—it's hard to stop eating.   Y/N

I sometimes "pig out" at meals.   Y/N

Interpretation: If you answered "yes" to any of the first six questions, you have a weight problem and you know it. If you answered "no" to the first six questions but did answer "yes" to two or more of the remaining questions, there's a good chance that you're overweight but may be in denial of it.

The Long-Term Consequences of Being Prediabetic and Overweight

Prediabetes, diabetes, and obesity are associated with an increased risk of developing many other health problems. You can lower your risk of suffering from these health problems by controlling your blood sugar and your weight.

Faster aging. Scientists regard diabetes as a type of accelerated aging. That's because normal age-related health problems occur earlier in life among people who have diabetes. For example, people with diabetes or prediabetes are more likely to develop heart disease or cancer at younger ages. If you want to live a long life, being prediabetic, diabetic, or overweight is not the way to do it.

People don't wake up one day to discover that they're suddenly diabetic. The progression from normal to prediabetic and then to diabetic typically occurs over many years. Furthermore, the slightest changes toward prediabetes are an ominous medical sign.

Heart disease. People with diabetes have four-times higher risk of incurring a heart attack compared with people who don't have diabetes.

Some of the Conditions Associated with Prediabetes, Diabetes, and Overweight

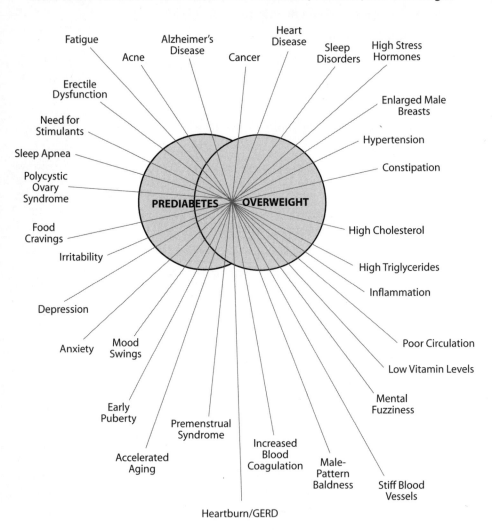

Prediabetes, diabetes, and overweight are associated with an increased risk of developing many other health problems. You can lower your risk by controlling your blood sugar and weight.

Here's another way of looking at your risk: let's say you work and socialize with sixteen people. If you're healthy, you have a one-in-sixteen chance of having a heart attack. If you're diabetic, your odds jump to one in four.

You don't have to be a full-blown diabetic to boost your risk of having a heart attack. Several studies have shown that modest elevations in blood sugar—within the normal range—can significantly increase your risk of suffering a heart attack. People with prediabetes or those who are overweight tend to have high levels of cholesterol, triglycerides, and inflammation—all are known risk factors for heart disease.

Elevated cholesterol. People who are prediabetic, diabetic, or overweight tend to have high levels of cholesterol, the "bad" low-density lipoprotein (LDL) cholesterol, and triglyceride levels, combined with low levels of the "good" high-density lipoprotein (HDL) cholesterol. This type of blood-fat profile is part of Syndrome X and is associated with an increased risk of developing heart disease. (For more information, see Jack's earlier book *Syndrome X.*)

High blood pressure. Hypertension is considered a leading risk factor for heart disease. Higher blood pressure leads to greater pounding of the blood vessels, kind of like strong waves crashing against a pier. This stress damages blood vessels. Research points to elevated insulin levels as the principal factor in hypertension.

Inflammation. Prediabetes, diabetes, and overweight boost the activity of the body's pro-inflammatory chemicals, such as interleukin-6 and C-reactive protein (CRP). Inflammation is now regarded as the underlying cause of heart disease. Basically, low-grade inflammation of the arteries leads to damage and sets the stage for cholesterol deposits. (For more information, see Jack's earlier book *The Inflammation Syndrome.*)

Low-grade infection. High blood-sugar levels interfere with the body's ability to fight bacterial infections. Doctors have known for more than a century that people with diabetes are especially susceptible to infections. In laboratory tests, high-sugar foods reduce the activity of white blood cells within minutes. Infections also promote inflammation.

Cancer. High insulin levels have been linked to breast, prostate, and colon cancers. Excess insulin seems to promote the growth of cancers. A study in the March 2007 issue of *Diabetes Care* reported that women with elevated blood-sugar levels were about 25 percent more likely to develop cancer. In addition, cancer patients often have symptoms of prediabetes.

Alzheimer's disease. There's strong evidence that prediabetes and

A Point to
Remember

Prediabetes, dia-
betes, and excess
weight increase
your risk of develop-
ing a large number
of serious diseases.

diabetes increase the risk of developing Alzheimer's disease. The mechanism may be related to
elevated blood-sugar levels or insulin resistance in
the brain. High levels of blood sugar also generate
dangerous molecules called free radicals, which
may damage both brain cells and blood vessels in
the brain.

Poor concentration. One of the classic signs of
diabetes is poor concentration, or feeling fuzzy
headed. This appears to be related to abnormally
high levels of blood sugar, which suppress orexins, a group of brain
chemicals that keeps our minds sharp and alert.

Mood swings. Moods often follow blood-sugar levels. Most people feel
contented after eating. When they get hungry, however, they can become
grumpy, impatient, irritable, angry, mean, and aggressive. People with
these changeable moods are often described as mercurial or Jekyll-and-
Hyde types. (For more information, see Jack's earlier book *The Food-
Mood Solution.*)

Kidney failure. High levels of blood sugar are toxic to the kidneys,
organs that help your body to filter out toxins. People with diabetes are
far more likely to suffer kidney failure, which is treated with surgery and
regular dialysis treatments.

Eye diseases. High levels of blood sugar make blood platelet cells
abnormally sticky, increasing the risk of blood clots. These clots are
especially serious in the tiny blood vessels of the eyes, where they can
lead to blindness. In addition, cataracts, glaucoma, and macular degen-
eration are strongly associated with glucose intolerance.

Nerve damage. People with diabetes have a very high risk of developing nerve damage, called neuropathy. This may lead to either pain or
numbness. In the case of numbness, diabetics cannot feel foot injuries,
which may become infected. A recent study found that people diagnosed with either carpal tunnel syndrome or Bell's palsy (characterized
by weakened or paralyzed facial muscles) are often prediabetic and will
be diagnosed with diabetes within ten years.

Sleep apnea. This condition entails a swelling of tissues in the back of
the mouth, leading to episodes of choking and interrupted breathing

during sleep. Severe snoring is really a form of sleep apnea. Being over-weight strongly predisposes people toward sleep apnea.

Erectile dysfunction. The inability to maintain an erection is a common complication of prediabetes and more so with full-blown diabetes. Erectile dysfunction may be a sign of more serious circulatory problems.

Early puberty. Although scientists have not figured out exactly why, a high-sugar diet often leads to early puberty in boys and girls. Today, adolescents start puberty at least one year earlier than adolescents did a century ago. It is very likely that high blood-sugar and insulin levels increase the activity of testosterone and estrogen.

Amputation. Because of blood vessel disease and circulatory problems, people with diabetes have a high risk of developing gangrene, necessitating amputation of fingers, toes, or an entire foot or leg.

Surgical complications. A study published in the April 2006 *Archives of Surgery* reported that people with diabetes had twice the risk of post-operative infections, compared with patients who did not have glucose-tolerance problems. This makes surgery far more dangerous for people who are prediabetic and diabetic.

Blood Sugar and Insulin: Understanding the Deadly Duo

Now we'll explain a little more about blood sugar and insulin, the two substances that play central roles in prediabetes, diabetes, and over-weight.

What You Need to Know about Blood Sugar

Blood sugar, or glucose, is the principal fuel of the body and the brain. Your body makes glucose by breaking down other types of sugar (such as table sugar), carbohydrates (such as pasta), and protein (such as meat and fish). Fats can serve as an alternate fuel source for most organs.

In nature, sugars and starches are almost always intertwined with fiber, the indigestible part of plants. The fiber in most vegetables and fruits and some whole grains slows the digestion of starches and sugars, leading to a gradual increase in blood sugar. This slow rise in blood sugar, followed by a moderate increase in insulin, is normal and healthy. Similarly, the digestion of protein results in very small increases in (and occasionally slight decreases) blood sugar. The more stable your blood sugar, the less likely you will experience hunger jags.

Pure sugars, however, such as sucrose and high-fructose corn syrups, are digested very quickly, leading to rapid increases in blood-sugar levels. Likewise, the starches in bread, pasta, pizza dough, muffins, bagels, and potatoes are also digested quickly. When blood-sugar levels shoot up, the body responds with a surge of insulin, which helps to lower blood-sugar levels. However, an insulin surge often reduces blood-sugar levels to *below* where they originally were, making people even hungrier. These extreme ups and downs in glucose and insulin are more likely to affect you than are more moderate changes in glucose and insulin levels.

When sharp blood-sugar swings occur day after day for many years, baseline (or fasting) blood-sugar levels gradually creep upward. The higher the blood sugar, the more likely it will start to *auto-oxidize* and generate hazardous molecules called free radicals. This auto-oxidation is a little like a chain reaction—one free radical can create another and another. The free radicals damage the body, speeding up the aging process and increasing your risk of developing heart disease and cancer. In fact, many of the complications of diabetes are related to high glucose levels and the free radicals they produce. (Antioxidants and certain vitamins, which we'll discuss in chapter 10, can neutralize free radicals.)

What You Need to Know about Insulin

Insulin is commonly regarded as the hormone that regulates blood-sugar levels, although it does far more than this. Biologically, it's one of the most ancient of all hormones.

In fact, insulin is an extremely potent anabolic hormone, meaning that it promotes the production of new tissue. It can stimulate the development of muscle, but high levels of insulin trigger a biological switch that turns off the production of muscle and switches on the production of fat, particularly around the belly. That's why insulin is considered the fat-storage hormone.

In addition, insulin helps convert blood sugar into triglycerides and then into body fat. Insulin also interferes with the breakdown of fat cells, so high insulin levels make it more difficult for you to lose weight.

Insulin resistance and high blood-sugar levels are the two trademarks of prediabetes and diabetes. But what exactly do we mean by insulin resistance? To explain, each time you eat a sugary or carbohydrate-rich food, your blood sugar surges. In response, your body releases insulin to help get rid of excess blood sugar.

The more your pancreas secretes insulin in an effort to control blood sugar, the less sensitive, or responsive, the rest of your body becomes to that insulin. Your body secretes still more insulin, and you become even less responsive to it. Insulin resistance develops when your body ignores what the insulin is trying to accomplish. Insulin levels continue to increase until your body's ability to make it wears out.

Although many of the complications of prediabetes and diabetes have been attributed to elevated blood sugar, high insulin levels actually seem to do far greater damage. Elevations in insulin precede increases in blood sugar by as much as fifteen years, leading to increases in belly fat, blood pressure, and blood fats. Sometimes doctors ask type 2 diabetic patients to inject themselves with insulin to control blood-sugar levels, but extra amounts of insulin boost their risk of developing heart disease and cancer.

Insulin also increases levels of cortisol, the body's principal stress hormone, and C-reactive protein, a promoter and a marker of inflammation. This relationship between insulin and CRP is significant for two reasons. One, inflammation aggravates many of the complications of diabetes, including kidney and eye disease. Two, inflammation is involved in every disease process, either causing or exacerbating symptoms and promoting the spread of the disease.

Three Must-Have Medical Tests

Three simple medical tests can clarify your risk of developing prediabetes, and several other tests may be helpful.

Fasting Glucose

Fasting glucose is part of nearly all conventional blood tests that patients undergo in the doctor's office and the hospital. It's based on the amount of glucose in a sample of blood taken in the morning, before you eat or drink anything except water.

If you've recently had blood tests, you can call your doctor's office to get a copy of your results. Your fasting blood sugar will be identified as "glucose." Our definitions of "better" and "best" glucose levels (see the following) are fairly strict compared with most doctors'.

Normal fasting glucose range: 65–99 mg/dl

Better fasting glucose range: 75–85 mg/dl

Best fasting glucose range: 80–82 mg/dl

Prediabetic fasting glucose range: 100–125 mg/dl

Diabetic fasting glucose range: 126 and above

There are two limitations to the fasting glucose test. First, the normal range (65–99 mg/dl) is far too wide. Minor increases within the norm can influence your long-term risk of developing diabetes and having a heart attack. One recent study found that young men with a fasting blood sugar of 87 mg/dl (well within the normal range) were far more likely to develop diabetes than were men whose fasting blood sugar was 81 mg/dl or less. Second, a normal fasting glucose test result can still miss a blood-sugar problem, but a fasting insulin test can usually ferret out less obvious blood-sugar problems.

Fasting Insulin

If your fasting glucose is between 65 and 99 mg/dl, your doctor may say your blood sugar is normal—but it may be a "false normal." Some people are very good at pumping out plenty of insulin, which will keep their glucose levels in the normal range. But high insulin, also known as hyperinsulinemia, is a smoking gun: it can increase your risk of developing prediabetes and diabetes by eight times!

As with fasting glucose, the normal range of fasting insulin—6 to 35 mcIU/ml—is too wide to be of any practical use. The higher your insulin, the harder your body is working to keep glucose levels down.

Identified early enough, elevated insulin is a red flag indicating prediabetes. Here are some better guidelines for interpreting your insulin
levels.

Normal fasting insulin range: 6–35 mcIU/ml

Better fasting insulin range: Less than 10 mcIU/ml

Best fasting insulin range: Less than 7 mcIU/ml

Prediabetic fasting insulin range: More than 11 mcIU/ml

Dangerous fasting insulin range: More than 25 mcIU/ml

As a person's glucose tolerance decreases—that is, as he or she
becomes more prediabetic and then diabetic—the body secretes more
insulin to control glucose levels. More insulin becomes necessary to
overcome the body's growing resistance to the normal activity of
insulin. After several years, the insulin resistance becomes so pronounced that glucose levels start to climb. That's why people with type
2 diabetes commonly have elevated levels of both insulin and glucose.

Your doctor may hesitate to measure your
insulin levels, and your insurer may be reluctant
to pay for it. But getting the test is in your own
best interest, so insist on it.

Your fasting insulin can also be combined with
your fasting glucose to calculate your homeostasis assessment model (HOMA) score, which
assesses your ability to make insulin and your
degree of insulin resistance. (See page 40 for more
on HOMA scores.)

> **A Point to Remember**
>
> A high fasting insulin level is a sign of pre-diabetes, even if your blood-sugar level appears normal.

Hemoglobin A$_{1c}$

This test, commonly abbreviated as HbA$_{1c}$ and called glycated hemoglobin, looks at how blood sugar has damaged proteins in your blood. In
doing so, the test provides a snapshot of your average glucose levels over
the previous six weeks. HbA$_{1c}$ levels are measured as a percentage,
using the symbol %.

Like fasting glucose and insulin, this test is very simple and reveals
what a single fasting glucose test might not. In a study of more than ten

thousand middle-age and elderly men and women, British researchers found that the risk of developing health problems increased when HbA_{1c} levels were above 5%, and the risk of having a heart attack increased by about 20 percent for each 1% rise in HbA_{1c} levels. In other words, a person with an HbA_{1c} of 6.0% was 20 percent more likely to have a heart attack compared with a person who had an HbA_{1c} of 5.0%. With an HbA_{1c} of 7.0%, a person was 42 percent more likely to suffer a heart attack.

Here is how you can interpret your HbA_{1c} test:

Normal HbA_{1c}: 4.5 to 5.7%

Best HbA_{1c}: Less than 5%

Prediabetic HbA_{1c}: 5.7 to 6.9%

Diabetic HbA_{1c}: 7% or higher

The HbA_{1c} test has certain advantages over a fasting glucose test. Sometimes, eating a lot of sugary foods the day before a fasting glucose test will throw off the results of the test. The HbA_{1c} provides your average blood sugar in recent weeks. An HbA_{1c} of 5.0% converts to 81 mg/dl average glucose, 5.2% to 87 mg/dl, 6.0% to 114 mg/dl, and 7.0% to 147 mg/dl.

Other Useful Medical Tests

Several additional tests may be helpful to you and your doctor, depending on your symptoms, medical history, and known risk factors for disease.

Triglycerides

Triglycerides are a type of blood fat and, like cholesterol, high levels are associated with an increased risk of developing heart disease. Elevated triglyceride levels usually reflect a diet that's high in refined sugar and carbohydrates. While levels above 150 mg/dl are generally considered only borderline high, they are strongly associated with prediabetes, especially when combined with overweight or acanthosis nigricans (a darkening of the skin on the neck, the groin, and the underarms). If you have a normal blood-sugar level but elevated triglycerides, ask your doctor to run further tests, such as fasting insulin and HbA_{1c}.

Normal triglycerides: 150 mg/dl or less

Best triglycerides: 100 mg/dl or less

Borderline elevated triglycerides: 150–199 mg/dl

High triglycerides: 200–499 mg/dl

Very high triglycerides: 500 mg/dl or above

A combination of elevated triglycerides and high levels of low-density lipoprotein (LDL) cholesterol (above 150 mg/dl) is an especially strong indicator of developing diabetes and heart disease risk. You can lower your triglyceride levels by cutting back on sugar and refined carbs, and LDL levels can be reduced by eating fewer trans fats (found in partially hydrogenated vegetable oils) and saturated fats (found in fatty meats).

Elevated levels of total cholesterol and LDL cholesterol, along with low levels of the high-density lipoprotein (HDL) cholesterol, also point to diets that are rich in refined sugarlike carbohydrates. We've focused on triglyceride levels here for the sake of simplicity. As your eating habits improve, however, your LDL cholesterol level will likely decrease, and your HDL cholesterol level will likely increase—both positive changes.

Glucose-Tolerance Test

Your doctor might ask you to take a glucose tolerance test over two to five hours. In this test, you'll have a blood draw before drinking a glucose solution, followed by additional measurements each hour. The glucose solution is icky sweet, and getting blood drawn every hour isn't a lot of fun.

As an alternative, some doctors measure their patients' fasting glucose in the morning, ask them to go to a restaurant and eat their typical breakfast, and then have them return to the office for more blood-sugar tests. The mix of sugar, carbs, and fats will increase glucose levels, which are measured after one, two, or more hours.

An increase or decrease of more than 50 mg/dl of glucose within any one-hour period points to glucose intolerance and prediabetes. Diabetes is diagnosed with a glucose level of 200 mg/dl or higher two hours after starting a glucose-tolerance test or eating breakfast.

HOMA

The HOMA (homeostasis assessment model) test is a calculation based on a patient's fasting glucose and fasting insulin levels. It determines the degree of insulin resistance (HOMA-IR) and the activity of pancreatic beta cells (%B), which manufacture insulin. You or your doctor can use a simple HOMA calculator to type in your fasting glucose and insulin levels. (The calculator can be found at www.dtu.ox.ac .uk/index.php.)

A normal HOMA-IR is 1.0, and a normal beta-cell function (%B) is 100 percent. This norm is based on a healthy person, of normal weight, thirty-five years of age or younger. A normal HOMA-IR and %B is worth targeting. Abnormal HOMA-IR levels are calculated based on variations from the norm.

A couple of examples convey the value of the HOMA calculation. A client of Jack's, Robert, had a fasting glucose of 85 mg/dl (normal) and a fasting insulin of 39 mcIU/ml (elevated). His HOMA-IR was calculated to be 4.7, pointing to severe insulin resistance and prediabetes. His %B was 320 percent, indicating very high beta-cell secretion of insulin to maintain normal glucose levels. His high level of insulin secretion will eventually wear out, leading to elevated glucose and diabetes.

A recent calculation of Jack's fasting glucose (82 mg/dl) and fasting insulin (4.9 mcIU/ml) found his HOMA-IR to be 0.6 and his %B to be 84. His below-normal HOMA-IR is exceptionally good (you could say better than normal), and his low %B indicates that he is not stressing his pancreas.

C-Reactive Protein

C-reactive protein (CRP) is both a marker and a promoter of inflammation. CRP levels can reach as much as 500 mg/dl in serious inflammatory diseases (such as rheumatoid arthritis) and trauma (life-threatening injuries).

In the late 1990s, Harvard Medical School researchers developed a more sensitive version of the test, called the high-sensitive C-reactive protein (hsCRP) test. This test identifies chronic low-grade inflammation that substantially increases the risk of developing heart disease and having a heart attack.

Elevated hsCRP levels are common in people who are overweight or have diabetes, and they point to low-grade inflammation. Other markers of inflammation, such as interleukin-6 and tumor necrosis factor alpha, are common in thin but flabby "preobese" people. People who eat a lot of sugary foods and refined carbohydrates also tend to have high levels of CRP.

Normal hsCRP: 0.11 mg/dl or less

Moderately elevated hsCRP: 0.12 to 0.19 mg/dl

High hsCRP: 0.20 to 1.50 mg/dl

Very high hsCRP: 1.51 to 3.7 mg/dl

Extremely high hsCRP: 3.8 mg/dl or higher

High levels of hsCRP can be reduced by losing weight, exercising, improving your glucose tolerance, eating more vegetables, using turmeric as a spice in your foods, taking vitamin E supplements, and reducing your consumption of sugary foods and refined carbs.

In this chapter, you've learned how to assess your likelihood of becoming prediabetic and overweight. By combining the quizzes and the information from medical tests, you and your physician will have a pretty clear grasp of your health. In the next chapter, we explain some of the dietary factors that set the stage for developing prediabetes and diabetes and becoming overweight.

2

Food Isn't What It Used to Be

I magine for a moment that you are a scientist who wants to make people overweight, prediabetic, and ultimately diabetic. There would be no better way than by feeding them the foods now eaten by most Americans.

To help you understand exactly how we—as individuals and as a society—make ourselves sick, let's review some basic principles of nutrition: the different types of nutrients in foods, how our society's eating habits have changed, and the foods that predispose you to developing prediabetes and becoming overweight.

What Exactly Are Nutrients?

What you eat (or don't eat) has the greatest bearing on your risk of becoming prediabetic, diabetic, and overweight. Eating habits are even more important than your genes, because your genes also depend on good nutrition.

Foods consist of complexes of many different nutrients, which fall into two general categories, macronutrients and micronutrients. Macronutrients refer to the larger constituents of our diets. Micronutrients are the smaller, but no less important, components of our diets.

Macronutrients

Macronutrients provide most of the volume, or calories, in our foods. They include protein, fats, carbohydrates, and sugars.

Protein. Protein is found in dairy products, fish, eggs, chicken, turkey, beef, pork, and other meats, as well as in beans, nuts, and seeds. A small amount of protein is also found in vegetables. During digestion, protein breaks down into chemicals called amino acids, which the body uses to make muscle, skin, internal organs, hormones, and chemicals that regulate our moods.

Fats. Many fats are essential for good health. They include two families of polyunsaturated fats (known as omega-3s and omega-6s) found in fish, green leafy vegetables, seeds, and nuts. Monounsaturated fats, which you get in avocados and in olive and macadamia nut oils, are also good for health. In addition, the body needs a small amount of saturated fat, found mostly in meats.

Carbohydrates. Carbohydrates generally refer to starches. Complex carbs have a larger chemical structure than that of simple carbs and sugars, and they are absorbed relatively slowly. High-fiber vegetables (e.g., leafy greens, tomatoes, broccoli, cauliflower) and high-fiber fruits (raspberries, blueberries, kiwi) are excellent sources of complex carbs.

In contrast, simple carbs are usually refined (such as by grinding, bleaching, or separating their constituents) to remove the fiber, resulting in an almost pure starch. Simple carbs are absorbed quickly, much like a sugar. White bread, white rice, pasta, pizza dough, and grits are examples of refined carbs. Potatoes contain a similar simple starch. Even most whole-grain products, including brown breads, have undergone significant processing and refining, resulting in absorption similar to that of sugars.

Sugars. Sugars are very simple carbs that consist of tiny and rapidly absorbed molecules. The two most common dietary sugars are sucrose (table sugar) and high-fructose corn syrup (a blend of fructose and glucose). The absorption of glucose and fructose in vegetables and fruits is slowed by fiber. The absorption of pure sugars, however, such as sucrose and high-fructose corn syrup, is very rapid, leading to sudden spikes in blood-sugar and insulin levels.

Micronutrients

Micronutrients rarely, if ever, provide calories. They usually refer to nutrients we need in relatively small amounts.

Vitamins. Vitamins are probably the most familiar micronutrients. They function as essential cofactors in the thousands of biochemical processes that occur in the body. They are needed to make, repair, and regulate our genes, and many of the B vitamins are involved in regulating blood-sugar and insulin levels.

Minerals. Minerals are also essential cofactors in biochemical processes, and some, such as calcium and magnesium, form part of the structure of our bones. Others, such as chromium, help to maintain normal insulin function.

Vitaminlike nutrients. Many vitaminlike nutrients are found in foods or made by the body in very small quantities. Vitaminlike nutrients include alpha-lipoic acid, coenzyme Q10, and antioxidants such as carotenoids and flavonoids.

How Our Foods Have Changed

The types of foods people eat have changed considerably over the years. Because of these changes, contemporary foods are richer in sugars and sugarlike carbs, significantly increasing people's risk of becoming prediabetic and overweight. These foods also contain relatively low levels of protective vitamins, minerals, vitaminlike nutrients, protein, healthy fats, and complex carbs.

The ancient diet of human beings consisted of whole foods, and this type of diet is what we're best suited for, biologically. In the distant past, nothing was refined or processed, and no foods came in boxes, cans, bottles, jars, or bags. There weren't any fast-food restaurants, fattening snacks, or rich desserts to tempt people. Our ancestors hunted for meat and gathered vegetables and plants. Prediabetes and overweight are major health problems today in large part because of a mismatch between our biological requirements for food and what we actually eat.

When did these dietary changes begin? They actually started thousands of years ago, but around 1900 the pace of food processing and refining accelerated, largely because of the industrialization of food processing. At that time, grain millers began to separate the wheat germ (seed) from its surrounding endosperm (consisting mostly of starch). With this change, whole-grain brown bread gave way to refined white flour and white bread. The more nutritious germ was often fed to livestock because they thrived on it, while people preferred the starchy portion.

Around the same time, millers also switched from stone to metal grinding wheels, enabling them to produce a finer and more powdery flour, resulting in a more sugarlike starch. Just a few years later, bleaching techniques were adopted to turn brown flour into white. The combination of refining and bleaching removed or destroyed much of the nutritional value of whole grains. Similar techniques were applied to the refining of sugars.

The consumption of more refined carbohydrates and sugar increased throughout the twentieth century. During the 1950s, fast foods (such as McDonald's) and convenience foods (then TV dinners, now microwave meals) grew in popularity. And by the 1970s and 1980s, large numbers of people were eating processed and refined foods, purchased either at the supermarket or in fast-food restaurants.

During the 1980s, food companies began to use high-fructose corn syrup to sweeten soft drinks, ice cream, and other foods. High-fructose corn syrup appears to be worse than plain old sugar in terms of its health effects. Food companies also started to use large amounts of trans fats (in the form of partially hydrogenated vegetable oils), which contribute to diabetes, overweight, and heart disease.

Another change during the 1980s was the popularity of low-fat and zero-fat diets. Such diets almost always were high-carb and high-sugar diets, with the additional carbs and sugar further propelling people toward prediabetes. Because of the combined effect of these changes, the average person's food consumption increased by several hundred calories daily over the 1980s and 1990s. All of these changes have heightened the risk of people developing prediabetes and becoming overweight. Similar trends have appeared wherever American soft drinks and fast foods have been marketed in Europe and Asia.

Changing Her Eating Habits, Gaining More Energy

Janet was overweight and complained about being tired all of the time. She never ate breakfast, thinking that would help her lose weight. At work, Janet had a "little taste" of doughnuts or cakes that her coworkers brought in, as well as coffee with sugar. For lunch, she got a burger or fried chicken and ate at her desk.

She usually began to feel drowsy about forty minutes after lunch, and she snacked on candies and soft drinks to perk up during the afternoon. At home after work, Janet usually heated a frozen dinner in the microwave, ate it, and often heated and ate a second one because she was so hungry. She then fell asleep on the sofa, woke up about 8 p.m., watched television, and went to bed around 11:30 p.m.

Janet's eating habits were a disaster, and she had difficulty improving them. Little by little, however, she made the attempt. She began to have an egg and a little fruit for breakfast, even though she worried that the calories and the fat in the egg would lead to more weight gain. To her surprise, she found that she had less interest in snacking in the morning. For lunch, she bought and ate a salad (with chicken, ham, or tuna) in a nearby park. Her energy levels were higher and she had no need for her normal afternoon snack.

At home, Janet made simple dinners with fresh chicken or fish and vegetables. No longer feeling wiped out after dinner, she watched television or read for a while, before going to sleep at 9:30 p.m. Now Janet regularly woke up earlier than in the past and felt energized enough to make a quick breakfast to start her day. She lost ten pounds in the first month after she changed her eating habits, and she continued to lose until she reached her target weight.

Calorie and Carb Alerts!

A sedentary man requires about 2,000 calories each day, and a sedentary woman needs about 1,600 calories daily. With calorie-packed fast foods and soft drinks, it's easy to consume practically all of these calories in a single meal. Today, the average adult American consumes almost 4,000 calories daily, most of them from sugar, sugarlike carbs, and unhealthy fats.

How can people possibly eat so many calories? It's easy, and we'll give you a couple of examples. A McDonald's Big Mac provides 560 calories (47 grams of sugars and carbs), a large order of fries has 570 calories (70 grams of carbs), and a Chocolate Triple Thick Shake has 580 calories (102 grams of sugars and carbs). At 1,710 calories, this one meal would provide more than a full day's calories for women and almost a full day's worth for men.

A slice of a Pizza Hut 12-Inch Super Supreme medium-size pan pizza has 330 calories (29 grams of carbs and sugars). Eat four of these small slices, which is easy, and you'll consume half of your daily calorie requirement. Eat the entire pizza, which many people do, and you'll consume 2,640 calories and 232 grams of carbs and sugars. Wash it down with a large (22-ounce) Mountain Dew, and you'll add 300 more calories and 85 grams of sugars and carbs. That's far more calories than most people need in a single day, and, nutritionally, they're low-quality calories.

Bigger Portions, More Snacking

Why are people now eating so much food? Part of the problem is that food portion sizes have increased immensely, enabling us to consume far more calories and carbohydrates each time we sit down to eat at home and in restaurants. Even dinner plates today are larger than they were in the 1950s.

In addition, people snack more often than they did in the past, and frequent snacking in itself can often be a sign of the up-and-down blood-sugar swings and food cravings that are characteristic of prediabetes. Because of larger portion sizes and more frequent snacking, it's easy to lose track of the huge amount of calories consumed in a meal or over the course of a day.

BARBARA'S STORY
Tackling Prediabetes

At forty-five, Barbara was prediabetic and on the fast track to developing full-blown diabetes. She was about forty pounds overweight, her fasting blood sugar was 116 mg/dl, and her fasting insulin was 28 mcIU/ml. Her body was pumping out plenty of insulin in an increasingly difficult effort to control her blood sugar. In addition, Barbara's triglycerides were very high at 220 mg/dl, and her total cholesterol was 290. Her "bad" low-density lipoprotein (LDL) cholesterol was also elevated at 190 mg/dl, and her "good" high-density lipoprotein (HDL) cholesterol was a low 25 mg/dl.

The good news was that Barbara was highly motivated. Her mother had died from complications of diabetes, and Barbara didn't want that to happen to her. She wanted to improve her health as much as possible with better eating habits and supplements, and she hoped to avoid taking medications.

A dietary analysis found that Barbara was eating a lot of refined sugar and carbs and relatively little protein and vegetables. Meanwhile, tests showed her to be low in vitamin B1 and chromium, magnesium, manganese, and zinc—all of which are nutrients involved in glucose and carbohydrate metabolism.

Barbara began to follow a diet that was high in healthy proteins, such as fish and chicken, as well as in vegetables. She also took a high-potency multivitamin, omega-3 fish oils, and vitamin and mineral supplements. She said she wasn't trying to "diet to lose weight," but she lost twenty pounds in three months and a total of forty pounds in six months. Barbara also began taking a brisk thirty-minute walk before eating her lunch.

Follow-up tests showed significant improvements. In addition to the weight loss, her fasting blood sugar was down to 87 mg/dl, and her fasting insulin was 9.5 mcIU/ml. Barbara's triglycerides, total cholesterol, and LDL cholesterol had decreased significantly, while her HDL cholesterol increased to 40 mg/dl. She was on the right track, and buoyed by her improvements, Barbara was motivated to stick with her regimen.

More than thirty years ago, the late Carlton Fredericks, Ph.D., observed that with people who are prediabetic or diabetic, larger amounts of sugar are needed to satisfy a sweet tooth. The situation is somewhat like a drug addiction in which larger amounts of the drug are needed to feel good. Conversely, when glucose tolerance improves, a person's sweet tooth becomes more sensitive, so less sugar provides a greater sense of sweetness.

Holiday Weight Gain Sticks with You

Researchers at the U.S. National Institutes of Health recently calculated that people consume about 25 percent more calories than usual around Thanksgiving and Christmas. On average, people gain a little more than one pound of weight during the holidays. But 20 percent of people gain between two and five pounds over the holidays, and 10 percent put on more than five pounds. In most cases, people do not lose this weight during the following spring or fall. It just adds up year after year.

Of course, these extra calories—think sugary and carb-rich foods—are above and beyond the regular huge portions that people eat on most days. Researchers have also found that people tend to eat substantially more on Fridays, Saturdays, Sundays, and celebratory days (e.g., at birthdays, retirement parties). On these days, people eat an average of 300 calories more than they do on other days.

The Hidden Calories and Carbs in Soft Drinks, Juices, and Coffee

Beverages now provide almost one-fourth of the calories Americans consume, and soft drinks alone account for 47 percent of the added sugar in the American diet. Yet relatively few people consider the calories from soft drinks, juices, or frothy frappucinos among the total number of calories they consume.

Huge Amounts of Sugar in Soft Drinks and Juices

A 12-ounce can of Coca-Cola Classic, like most other soft drinks sweetened with high-fructose corn syrup, contains the equivalent of ten teaspoons of sugars. If you drink just one can of regular Coke, Pepsi, or Mountain Dew a day, all that sugar can pack on fifteen pounds over the course of a year. That alone can put you on the fast track to prediabetes.

Consider soft drinks a source of stealth calories. Serving sizes have increased substantially over the years, contributing to a growth in waist sizes. During the first half of the twentieth century, Coke and other soft drinks were sold either as fountain drinks or in 6.5-ounce bottles. In the 1950s, Coca-Cola and other companies increased bottle sizes to 10 and 12 ounces, practically doubling the number of calories per serving.

Incredibly, 12-ounce cans are now the pygmies of the supermarket soft drink aisle. Two-quart (64-ounce) bottles dominate supermarket shelves and are also sold as Double Gulp soft drinks at 7-Eleven convenience stores. Granted, not everyone drinks an entire two-quart bottle each day, but many people do—or they consume the lion's share of it while sitting at their desks or driving their cars.

A two-quart bottle of Coca-Cola Classic contains 800 calories and almost a half-pound (216 grams) of sugars. Tropicana Lemonade, which might sound healthier, provides practically the same quantity of sugars. If you drink the entire bottle, you get far more sugar than you would in a glucose-tolerance test at your doctor's office.

Orange Crush and Sunkist hold the dubious distinction of containing the largest quantities of sugars in soft drinks. A two-quart bottle of Orange Crush weighs in at 960 calories and more than a half-pound of sugars (272 grams). That's about half the daily calories most people need but without any redeeming nutritional value. Sunkist

---

QUICK TIP

What's the Problem with Just a Few Sugar Calories or Simple Carbs?

The problem is that a few sugar calories and simple carbs here and there quickly add up to hefty amounts. It's best to stick with the very small amounts of natural sugar and carbs found in fruits and vegetables and to avoid all types of added sugar, such as sucrose and high-fructose corn syrup.

orange-flavored soft drinks are even worse. A two-quart bottle of Sunkist contains 1,040 calories and almost two-thirds of a pound (280 grams) of sugars.

A similar-size bottle of Ocean Spray Cranberry Juice Cocktail, which many people believe to be healthy, contains 1,040 calories and, like soft drinks, more than a half-pound of sugars (264 grams), nearly all of it coming from high-fructose corn syrup and not from cranberries. Even worse, a two-quart bottle of Welch's 100% Grape Juice contains 1,360 calories and almost three-quarters of a pound (320 grams) of sugars. It doesn't matter whether these are natural or added sugars—they come with virtually no other nutritional value.

Many so-called healthy drinks and juices aren't any better. An 8-ounce can of Ensure contains 250 calories (50 of them from fat), 18 grams of sugars, and 22 grams of other carbs. Two quarts add up to 2,000 calories (400 of them from fat), 144 grams of sugars, and 176 grams of other refined carbs. A 32-ounce bottle of R. W. Knudsen Just Pomegranate contains 600 calories and 144 grams of sugars, which, ounce for ounce, is worse than any soft drink.

In 2006, PepsiCo, the corporate parent of such companies as Pepsi-Cola and Frito-Lay, introduced Fuelosophy, a line of fruit-flavored smoothies geared to the health food market. Fuelosophy drinks have the same amount of sugars as an equal quantity of regular Pepsi but almost twice the calories.

The calorie- and sugar-rich Frappucino beverages from Starbucks are nothing more than caffeinated dessert drinks. A Venti-size (20-ounce) Banana Coconut Frappucino with whipped cream packs 730 calories—about one half of a woman's daily caloric requirement—and a quarter-pound (119 grams) of sugars. A Tazo Iced Green Tea Latte might sound healthier, but the Venti (24-ounce) size has 350 calories and 51 grams of sugars.

Sugar-Free Soft Drinks May Be Bad, Too

It sounds incredible, but sugar-free soft drinks and artificial sweeteners may be no better than sugary soft drinks.

Researchers have noted that people who consume two or more cans of either regular or diet soft drinks daily are about 50 percent more likely to become overweight or obese compared with people who do not consume soft drinks. It's not clear why sugar-free soft drinks would also lead to weight gain, but we have our suspicions. When people consume diet drinks, they may believe they can afford to indulge in calorie- and carb-rich foods, such as pizza.

The Complicity of Food Companies

The makers of processed foods and fast-food companies are in business to make a profit. We have no problem with companies making money,

> **QUICK TIP**
>
> **What Are High-Glycemic Foods?**
>
> High-glycemic foods trigger a sharp rise in blood-sugar levels, mainly because their sugar and starches are so quickly absorbed. High-glycemic foods include sugary soft drinks, candy bars, rice cakes, and potatoes.

as long as they do so ethically. However, we question the ethics of companies that develop, market, and sell foods that promote obesity, prediabetes, and diabetes.

Whenever controversies about eating habits make it to newspapers and the evening news, the food companies' public relations staffs and lobbyists typically say that their products are fine when consumed as part of a healthy balanced diet. They tend to blame the alarming rate of obesity and diabetes on individual food choices and inadequate exercise. The truth is that these companies are not passive participants in this modern health debacle. They aggressively promote unhealthy foods that are designed around sugars, sugarlike carbs, and trans fats and then shrug off any responsibility for contributing to obesity and prediabetes.

For many years, companies have had lucrative deals with public schools to stock vending machines with sugary soft drinks and high-sugar snacks. Although these companies are now withdrawing some of their high-calorie beverages and snacks from schools because of public pressure, we fear that the damage has already been done.

In the United States, the giant fast-food and soft drink companies compete for increased sales using marketing plans that resemble military battle plans. With the U.S. fast-food and soft drink markets now largely saturated, the giant food companies have worked to open new markets in Europe, Asia, and Central and South America where they can make greater financial gains.

The companies have succeeded in selling more and making more money—getting fat financially by making people fat and unhealthy. That's no better than how the cigarette companies marketed their products.

3

Dangers That Lurk beyond Calories and Carbs

People now consume far greater quantities of calories, sugars, and sugarlike carbohydrates than they did just a couple of generations ago, and this increase is one reason why many more people are now overweight and prediabetic. But several other factors exacerbate the situation and propel people toward developing prediabetes and becoming overweight.

Food Addictions: Why You Can't Stop Eating

Many people have a history of being yo-yo dieters. They have trouble sticking with a diet for more than a few weeks, let alone adhering to lifelong changes in eating habits. This on-a-diet, off-a-diet pattern illustrates the sheer power of food addictions. To improve your eating habits, you may have to confront the demon of food addictions.

Most food addictions involve cravings for foods that are loaded with sugar or refined carbohydrates, such as bread, chips, pretzels, candies, ice cream, chocolate, soft drinks, and pizzas. (We just can't picture many people sitting in front of the television with overwhelming cravings for salmon and broccoli.) In fact, simply thinking of a favorite food or smelling fries can trigger the secretion of digestive juices, which in turn leads to hunger pangs and cravings for those foods. There is often a psychological component as well: eating may be a source of comfort, a cure for boredom, or just something to keep your hands or mouth busy while you watch a movie or television. Whatever the reason, food addicts just can't stop eating.

The idea that food and drug addictions share many common features is not all that far-fetched. Considerable research has found similar types of brain activity in people who are overweight and those who are drug addicts. Both food and stimulant drugs, such as cocaine and methamphetamines, rapidly boost levels of the neurotransmitter dopamine in the brain. Dopamine is the brain's principal pleasure chemical—the ultimate upper, so to speak.

Economic factors can reinforce food addictions. Sugary and carb-rich foods are cheap and filling, but they make people hungrier—that is, in need of another "hit." Food companies and restaurants aggressively market sugary and carb-rich foods because they're cheap to make and very profitable, and the more people eat, the greater the profits. In contrast, protein is more expensive and it makes people less hungry, which means the food companies and the restaurants don't sell as much of it.

How do food addictions develop? We have several explanations.

First, blood-sugar swings, with their bouts of low blood sugar, lead to an eating pattern that strongly resembles an addiction cycle. Periods of low blood sugar can feel like drug withdrawal, and people frequently respond by eating whatever quickly boosts their blood sugar, typically a sugary or high-calorie snack. But as with drug addictions, such fixes create a need for increasingly frequent and calorie-rich fixes. Whether the problem is sugars, carbs, or coffee, the food addict needs more of the fix more often to avoid feeling withdrawal symptoms.

Second, if you have regular food cravings for specific foods, such as for bread or ice cream, your addiction has an even stronger resemblance to drug addiction. Foods containing wheat and dairy are two of the most common addictions. Both wheat and dairy foods contain trace amounts of naturally occurring opioids. Although these opioids are not in large-enough quantities to create a high, they likely help to cement certain food addictions. When we give speeches and talk about food addictions, one or two people invariably come up afterward to say they

MELINDA'S STORY
Overcoming a Soft Drink Addiction

Melinda, in her late forties, had long suffered from chronic fatigue syndrome, but she had enough enthusiasm and nutritional support to keep the disease from dominating her life. The one nutritional problem she could never seem to address was her love of soft drinks.

She was, in fact, addicted to soft drinks and for most of her life had consumed about three cans daily. Dr. Ron explained that each can contained about ten teaspoons of sugar, adding up to about 80 pounds of sugar a year. But Dr. Ron's message never really seemed to register with Melinda. After all, she once said, "It was only a few cans of pop."

At a recent annual appointment, Dr. Ron noted that Melinda had gained fifteen pounds and her blood pressure was high for the first time. Both changes are signs of prediabetes. With a family history of diabetes and stroke, Melinda sighed. She knew it was finally time for a change.

Making the change was not easy, and that's often the case with food addictions. Melinda switched to diet soft drinks and, over the next year, weaned herself off them completely. It was only when she stopped consuming all soft drinks that she started to lose weight and her blood pressure decreased. As a side benefit of the change, Melinda realized that her energy levels had improved.

---

couldn't ever imagine not eating bread or some other favorite food. That immediately tells us a lot about their food addictions.

Third, food addictions are commonly intertwined with food allergies, or sensitivities. (Traditional markers of allergies are not always present, so it often helps to look for other indicators.) In this view of food allergies, developed largely by the late Theron Randolph, M.D., regular consumption of the problematic foods can result in symptoms that mimic almost any type of illness, including aches and pains and fuzzy thinking.

Some evidence indicates that food allergies release endorphins, the body's own family of painkillers. People may become addicted to both the endorphins and the foods that trigger their release. People can be allergically addicted to healthy foods, not only to junk foods, with the problematic food usually being a person's favorite food.

Fourth, alcohol is a common food addiction, and alcoholics who crave specific types of alcoholic beverages may have an allergy-addiction to the grain or the vegetable that particular beverage is made from. In addition, excess consumption of alcohol may damage the gut wall. The consequence, known as "leaky gut syndrome," may allow undigested proteins to enter the bloodstream and trigger immune reactions.

Fifth, people can become addicted to a food's texture and the act of chewing that food. Some food textures are particularly addictive, such as sticky candies, popcorn, potato chips, pretzels, nuts, cookies, and ice cream. In sum, there are a great many reasons why people can become addicted to food—and why they can't stop eating. The inability to deal with food addictions is often why people cannot stay on a healthy diet.

The More You Eat, the Hungrier You Get

You might think that the more you eat, the less hungry you'd feel, but just the opposite happens. David Ludwig, M.D., of Harvard University, has shown that the blood-sugar swings that follow the consumption of sugary foods and refined carbohydrates trigger more frequent bouts of hunger, leading to greater food consumption and weight gain.

Part of the problem is that the fast foods, the convenience foods, and the junk foods contain large amounts of "high-glycemic" carbohydrates—another way to describe sugar and sugarlike refined carbohydrates. High-glycemic foods trigger a quick spike in blood sugar, followed by a surge of insulin, which causes blood sugar to fall lower than where it was before you ate. This means you get hungrier a little while after eating.

The More "Energy" Foods and Drinks You Have, the More Tired You Get

We've all been taught that sugar-rich foods are a quick source of energy, so it's no surprise that we often reach for sugary foods or beverages to perk up. But do you ever feel that the energy boost is short lived?

The late Hugh D. Riordan, M.D., whom we knew and worked with, believed that many people end up overeating because they keep trying to increase their energy levels. We think he made a profound point, and research has since shown that so-called energy foods tend to leave people feeling more tired, not energized.

As one example, British researchers reported in 2006 that people who consumed energy drinks, which contained hefty amounts of sugar and a little caffeine, did not feel more energized. Instead, the energy drinks slowed their reaction times, suggesting that the drinks made them more fuzzy and tired.

Many candy bars, in both supermarkets and health food stores, are marketed for their energy-boosting benefits. Nearly all of them contain various sugars, which would place them high on the glycemic index. They may temporarily boost blood-sugar and energy levels, but they also lead to a subsequent plummeting of blood-sugar levels. For all practical purposes, most of these energy bars are just another type of candy bar, and energy drinks are a soft drink that most people could do without.

How Do the Glycemic Index and the Glycemic Load Fit In?

To appreciate the effect of refined sugar and carbohydrates on your body, it helps to understand a little about the *glycemic index* and the *glycemic load*.

Both terms are rankings of how quickly sugar- and carb-containing foods get absorbed and boost blood-sugar levels. High-glycemic foods (such as sugary soft drinks, candy bars, rice cakes, and potatoes) trigger a sharp increase and a subsequent drop in blood-sugar levels. In contrast, low-glycemic foods (such as fresh vegetables) are absorbed slowly, resulting in more moderate increases in blood sugar.

For example, instant rice and corn flakes have extremely high rankings on the glycemic index, meaning that their effect on blood sugar is almost exactly that of pure glucose. Rice cakes, a staple for many dieters, have a glycemic index ranking of 110, which is 10 percent higher than pure glucose. Baked potatoes, another favorite food of dieters, are almost as bad. When dieters feel hungry most of the time, it's often because they're eating too many high-glycemic foods, which creates a blood-sugar roller coaster.

Some foods have extremely low rankings in the glycemic index and the glycemic load, meaning they have a negligible effect on blood-sugar levels. Broccoli has no effect, so it ranks as zero on both the glycemic index and the glycemic load. Peanuts have a low ranking on the glycemic index and have almost no effect on glycemic load. Carrots have a fairly high ranking on the glycemic index, but they are very low on the glycemic load, so a serving is not usually a problem. As a general rule, protein has little effect on blood-sugar levels and therefore little impact on the glycemic index and the glycemic load.

What's Wrong with the Glycemic Index and the Glycemic Load?

The glycemic index and the glycemic load have become popular references for people who are trying to lose weight and prevent diabetes. Many physicians and dietitians now recommend that their patients eat low-glycemic foods, but we see four key drawbacks to relying too much on the glycemic index and the glycemic load.

First, checking every food's ranking on the glycemic index can be as much of a hassle as counting calories and carbs. Many people just don't have the time to precisely calculate the glycemic values of foods or to figure out the average glycemic index of a multifood meal, which is what nearly everyone eats. Because such calculations become a chore, many people stop looking up the glycemic index of foods, just as they previously stopped counting calories and carbs.

Second, and perhaps more important, low-glycemic foods are not necessarily nutritious or healthy. For example, fettuccini, spaghetti, ice cream, and M&M peanut candies are relatively low on the glycemic index; however, they are not as nutritious as baked salmon and steamed vegetables.

Third, it's all too easy to overindulge in unhealthy low-glycemic foods, driven by the idea that they're healthy. Worse, as you increase portion sizes, the food's ranking on the glycemic index and glycemic load increases.

Fourth, glycemic responses to foods are highly individual. People with prediabetes are especially sensitive to carbs and sugars and tend to have strong reactions. For example, they may have high-glycemic responses to moderate-glycemic foods.

If you stick mostly to the healthy foods we recommend—namely, fish, chicken, lean meats, and a lot of vegetables—you'll automatically eat nutritious and low-glycemic foods. Better yet, you'll do so without having to look up foods and count numbers. We'll explain more about which foods to eat in chapter 4.

> **A Point to Remember**
>
> Foods low on the glycemic index are not necessarily healthy foods. Before you buy a low-glycemic food, consider whether it is actually nutritious.

Sometime a Calorie Is More Than a Calorie

You've heard the mantra that nearly every nutrition expert preaches: a calorie is a calorie. To lose weight, according to this line of thinking, people have to burn more calories than they consume. A calorie is a unit of energy, and your body burns calories for fuel much the way a car burns gasoline.

Many dieters, however, know that the calorie-is-a-calorie idea just isn't true. Their personal experiences tell them that they can gain several pounds of weight after eating a small quantity of, let's say, chocolate or pizza. But the average dieter doesn't have the scientific background to argue with the calorie-is-a-calorie experts.

The calorie-is-a-calorie approach is based, scientifically, on the first law of thermodynamics, which is an underpinning of chemistry and physics. The first law of thermodynamics is essentially about the amount of energy going into a system being equal to the amount of energy being released. To lose weight according to this line of thinking, a person must burn more energy (calories) than he or she consumes.

Yet tantalizing scientific evidence now indicates that some types of calories do count for more, and some people are more sensitive than others to the effect of these calories. Eugene J. Fine, M.D., and Richard D. Feinman, Ph.D., have pointed out that the second law of thermodynamics comes into play with living, breathing people. This law notes that there is an inherent inefficiency in all biological and biochemical processes. In other words, people burn energy less efficiently than cars do.

For example, people who are prediabetic or diabetic, or those who have been overweight for many years, don't burn calories very efficiently. Instead, they do an exceptional job of storing these calories as body fat. They're able to make more body fat out of fewer calories, compared with people who aren't overweight.

A Point to Remember

Some people are especially sensitive to sugar and carbohydrate calories. Maybe you are.

This is a controversial view, but we agree that some calories, in a manner of speaking, weigh more than other calories. People with prediabetes often have difficulty losing weight on low-fat, high-carb diets. Instead, they are more likely to lose weight on low-carb, high-protein diets. The reason is that people with prediabetes are extremely sensitive to sugar and carbohydrate calories. They do better with protein, which does not trigger a strong glucose response.

Interestingly, people who are overweight but not prediabetic tend to lose more weight on high-carb but low-calorie diets. The long-term problem, however, is that high-carb diets will eventually cause prediabetes, at which point these people will do better on a low-carb, high-protein diet.

The Two Most Dangerous Food Additives

Two specific food additives may be largely responsible for the increasing numbers of people who are overweight, obese, prediabetic, and diabetic. These additives are *high-fructose corn syrup* and *trans fats*;

the latter are found in *partially hydrogenated vegetable oils*. Most processed and packaged foods—those sold in boxes, cans, bottles, and jars—contain one or both of these additives. We list many of these foods in chapter 6.

High-Fructose Corn Syrup: Worse Than Sugar

Some people think of fructose as "fruit sugar" and regard it as healthy. In fact, many diabetic specialists and dietitians consider fructose a safe sugar for people with diabetes. Nothing could be further from the truth.

It's true that fruit contains fructose but in very small amounts. Nearly all of the fructose that people consume comes from processed corn sugars, which are added during the manufacture of packaged foods. Furthermore, the amount of fructose consumed has grown substantially in recent years.

From about 1910 through the early 1980s, the daily per capita consumption of carbohydrates (mostly starches) in the United States decreased from about 1.1 pounds to just over three-fourths of a pound. Since the 1980s, however, carbohydrate consumption has returned to the earlier level, but high-fructose corn syrup (a blend of sugars) accounts for nearly all of the increase.

Between 1980 and 2004, the average U.S. resident's intake of all sugars increased by almost one-fifth, from 120 to 141 pounds per year. Consumption of sucrose (ordinary white table sugar) decreased from about 84 to 62 pounds, while that of corn sugars increased from about 35 pounds to a little more than 78 pounds per year. Most of that increase pertained to high-fructose corn syrup, which jumped from 19 pounds to almost 60 pounds per person annually. That's more than 300 percent!

Until the use of high-fructose corn syrup became widespread, sucrose was the most common sweetener used in prepared foods and beverages, including soft drinks and pastries. Sucrose is a single molecule, which breaks down during digestion into equal parts (50:50) of glucose and fructose. Most of the high-fructose corn syrup on the market is actually a blend of two sugars: 55 percent fructose and 45 percent glucose. Fructose is also sweeter than sucrose or glucose, so foods made with high-fructose corn syrup taste much sweeter than those made with other sugars. Because of these and other characteristics, high-fructose corn syrup has largely replaced sucrose in soft drinks, candies, and pastries.

But because high-fructose corn syrup is a blend of fructose and glucose, it is metabolized differently from sucrose. More than forty years ago, the British researcher John Yudkin, M.D., Ph.D., found that the health effects of fructose were far worse than those of either glucose or sucrose, and recent research has confirmed and expanded on his findings.

Fructose bypasses the body's normal means of metabolizing sugar, and, in doing so, it is more "lipogenic" than glucose. This means it is more likely to be converted to various types of fat, and the growing prevalence of overweight and obesity correlates with the increase in consumption of high-fructose corn syrup. Fructose also increases blood levels of triglycerides, the "bad" low-density lipoprotein form of cholesterol, and the "very bad" very-low-density lipoprotein form of cholesterol. Furthermore, it raises blood pressure, which is associated with overweight and diabetes.

Some evidence indicates that fructose and high-fructose corn syrup have a more pronounced effect than do glucose and sucrose on taste receptors, imprinting both the tongue and the brain with a stronger desire for sweet foods throughout life. There is also evidence that fructose and high-fructose corn syrup modify the brain's appetite-regulating centers. Fructose decreases levels of leptin, a hunger-suppressing hormone, and it boosts levels of ghrelin, a hunger-stimulating hormone— creating a double-whammy that fosters more eating and weight gain.

As if that were not enough, fructose actually promotes diabetes. It reduces glucose tolerance, interferes with normal insulin function, increases insulin levels, promotes insulin resistance, and increases C-peptide levels (another marker of insulin resistance). Fructose is not safe for diabetics—or anyone else.

Trans Fats: An Ever-Present Danger

Trans fats are found in partially hydrogenated vegetable oils and shortening and foods made with these products. Shortening consists of almost one-fifth trans fats, and some brands of margarine contain almost one-fourth trans fats. The oils used to cook French fries and fried chicken in the United States consist of about 40 percent trans fats, and the amount increases when the cooking oil is heated. Trans fats now account for about 7.5 percent of the fat calories consumed in the United States, and the average American eats nearly five pounds of trans fats each year.

Partially hydrogenated vegetable oils and trans fats are produced when food manufacturers pump hydrogen atoms into soybean, cottonseed, and other vegetable oils. These artificial fats thicken foods, create a buttery texture, and extend shelf life. There is no safe level of intake, and they remain in foods solely as a convenience to food processors, fast-food restaurants, and restaurant chefs.

Researchers seem most concerned about how trans fats raise levels of the bad form of cholesterol and lower the good form, but the effects of trans fats are far more sinister. They do much of their damage by interfering with enzymes called desaturases and elongases, which are necessary for normal fat metabolism, and some evidence suggests that trans fats may alter normal gene activity. Essentially, trans fats fundamentally change how the body metabolizes other fats, leading to overweight and obesity.

Trans fats interfere with normal insulin function, reducing its ability to transport and burn glucose. They increase insulin resistance and raise blood levels of triglycerides. Researchers at Wake Forest University School of Medicine, in Winston-Salem, North Carolina, reported that trans fats increase insulin resistance, a hallmark of both prediabetes and diabetes. Even modest amounts of trans fats (less than what the average American currently consumes) are associated with an almost 40 percent increase in the risk of developing diabetes!

The researchers at Wake Forest University found that feeding trans fats (in amounts comparable to what people eat in fried foods) to monkeys led to a gain of 7.2 percent more body weight over six years. That's equivalent to about an 11-pound increase for a 150-pound person. Furthermore, monkeys consuming the trans fats had 30 percent more belly fat. In contrast, monkeys that consumed olive oil had only a 1.8 percent increase in their body weight.

Trans fats set the stage for a variety of health problems associated with overweight, prediabetes, and diabetes. Because of the way they modify fat metabolism, trans fats promote inflammation, a factor in almost every disease process. They increase the production of harmful molecules known as free radicals, which play a role in virtually every disease process. Trans fats also reduce blood vessel tone and flexibility, which ends up stiffening blood vessels and reducing circulation. The same mechanism seems to interfere with how men gain erections, so trans fats are likely involved in causing erectile dysfunction.

A New Fat That's Worse Than Trans Fats

Just when we thought that trans fats were the most dangerous of all food additives, a new type of fat concoction started to gain momentum in restaurants and packaged foods in early 2007. These fats are called interesterified fats, and food companies and restaurants have looked to them as a replacement for trans fats. But according to a study in the journal *Nutrition & Metabolism*, they're even more dangerous than trans fats!

> **A Point to Remember**
>
> Avoid all foods containing trans fats, shortening, and partially hydrogenated vegetable oils. These ingredients may not be identified in restaurants, so avoid all fried foods and be wary of prepared salad dressings.

Like trans fats, interesterified fats lower the "good" high-density lipoprotein cholesterol, which alters the ratios among blood fats and increases the risk of heart disease. But in a four-week study, the interesterified fats also raised the subjects' fasting blood sugar by 20 percent and their post-meal blood sugar by 40 percent, in comparison with saturated fats! These changes led the researchers to observe that interesterified fats made the subjects prediabetic in one month.

To identify interesterified fats on food packages, look for the phrases "interesterified soybean oil," "interesterified vegetable oil," "fully hydrogenated oil," "high in stearic acid," or "stearate rich" in the ingredient list on food labels.

An Advantage to Natural Fats

Calorie for calorie, you're less likely to gain weight if you consume a lot of the "healthy fats," particularly fish oil, olive oil, and macadamia nut oil. You're more likely to gain weight if you eat a lot of trans fats, vegetable oils, and saturated fats.

In experiments, researchers fed mice diets containing the same amounts of vegetable oils, saturated fats, or fish oils. Mice eating fish oils remained the leanest, whereas those eating the most vegetable oils gained the greatest amount of weight, even more than the mice eating saturated fats. Other studies have found that laboratory animals that consumed monounsaturated fats (such as olive oil) were less likely to gain weight, compared with mice that ate the same number of calories in saturated fats.

Human studies show substantial weight-loss benefits with the addition of omega-3 fish oils. Furthermore, the omega-3s improve glucose tolerance and reduce both insulin and triglyceride levels. The omega-3 fats play important roles in maintaining normal glucose tolerance, and high levels of vegetable oils and trans fats interfere with their normal activity. We'll explain more about the benefits of the omega-3 fish oils in chapter 10.

> **A Point to Remember**
>
> Trans fats, soybean oil, and saturated fats appear to increase body fat. Fish oils and olive oil may help to keep people slim.

Skipping Breakfast Makes Blood Sugar Worse and Contributes to Weight Gain

Many people skip breakfast, believing that it helps to reduce their caloric intake and blood sugar. But skipping breakfast actually has the opposite effect. It increases insulin resistance, the cornerstone of prediabetes and full-blown diabetes, and people more than make up the calories later in the day.

Two important studies demonstrated the benefits of eating a healthy breakfast on prediabetes, hunger, and overweight. In one, researchers fed subjects a variety of breakfasts. They found that high-fiber foods and slow-digesting carbohydrates led to improvements in blood sugar in less than one day.

In the other study, eating a protein-containing breakfast yielded even greater benefits. Researchers fed overweight women one of two breakfasts. The first consisted of scrambled eggs and toast, and the second was a bagel, cream cheese, and low-fat yogurt. Women eating the eggs for breakfast had a greater feeling of fullness for several hours. In fact, the breakfast was so satisfying that at lunchtime, the women ate almost one-fourth fewer calories.

The benefits didn't stop there. Over the next day and a half, the women who began their day with eggs each ate 420 fewer calories. If they had maintained that lower calorie intake over the course of a year, they each would have lost close to thirty pounds of weight.

Genetic Susceptibilities for Overweight and Prediabetes

Genes form the biological blueprint that governs how your body processes nutrients for energy, growth, and fighting disease. Years ago, scientists theorized that people inherited a "thrifty gene" that enabled them to store calories—that is, to get fat—during times of plenty, with the idea being that people could draw on that fat reserve during famines.

The thrifty gene idea might work for bears hibernating over the winter, but it doesn't seem to be relevant to people. Overweight people can die of starvation just as quickly as skinny people, so storing body fat offers no real biological advantage. In fact, the scientists who originally proposed the thrifty gene idea have since abandoned it, although the idea still has some adherents.

For the most part, the genetic link between genes and obesity remains murky. Since 1994, more than fifty genes have been linked to obesity; however, none of them is considered the arbiter of a person's weight. Likewise, although a few genes have been associated with diabetes, none seems to influence the risk of developing diabetes in the majority of people.

A better argument can be made for modern foods being incompatible with our ancient genes. Some researchers have described soft drinks, breads, cereals, pastas, and other processed and refined foods as being "genetically unknown foods." In other words, they give the wrong cues to our genes, increasing the risk of disease. Faced with large quantities of genetically unfamiliar nutrients—sugar, sugarlike carbs, and trans fats—our genes respond inappropriately, making us overweight and prediabetic.

HAROLD'S STORY
The Side Benefits of Losing Weight

Harold was a long-distance truck driver in his midfifties. He had spent most of his life driving across all forty-eight states, eating at truck stops, and sleeping in the cab of his truck. Harold enjoyed seeing the country, but he admitted that sometimes the boredom of the road got to him. He commented that the life of a truck driver sucked.

His age, deadlines, financial pressures, long hauls, and junk-food diet left him feeling trapped by his lifestyle. He knew he could not easily change careers. Over the last five years, Harold had gained more than fifty pounds, had developed severe hypertension (200/110 mmHg), and had been diagnosed with fibromyalgia, a condition characterized by extreme fatigue and achy muscles. "Sure, I'm overweight—who wouldn't be with this damn lifestyle!" he said.

Harold felt boxed in, and it wasn't clear that his lifestyle would allow him to make substantial improvements. To our pleasant surprise, though, he began to follow a protein-rich, low-carb eating plan. He felt better, lost some weight, and his blood pressure began to decrease. The pain from his fibromyalgia lessened, and his mood and outlook toward life improved significantly. Harold still has a ways to go, but he has made improvements and has started seeing the results.

The Stress Connection to Overweight and Prediabetes

Stress is often ignored as a factor in overweight and prediabetes. Exactly how does stress contribute to these health problems?

When people feel stressed, their eating habits almost always slide. Think about your own habits: when you're stressed, you're more likely to delay or skip meals, later opting for foods or snacks that are rich in sugars and sugarlike carbs, as well as beverages loaded with sugar and caffeine. These foods and beverages create a blood-sugar roller coaster, and they displace more nutritious foods that protect against weight problems and prediabetes.

Bad as that is, the damage gets worse. The breakdown of carbohydrates depends on a family of enzymes called dehydrogenases. The more sugar and carbs you eat, the more dehydrogenases your body must make. Dehydrogenases depend on vitamin B1, so eating a lot of sugar and carbs increases your requirements for this vitamin. Yet sugary foods and sugarlike carbs contain little of the vitamin. As a result, you are more likely to develop signs of a vitamin B1 deficiency, including mental fuzziness and confusion.

There's still more. Stress also increases the secretion of insulin and cortisol, the body's principal long-acting stress hormone. Both hormones work together to promote the formation of belly fat, contributing to both overweight and prediabetes. Stress also triggers the release of a variety of inflammatory compounds, including interleukin-6, which further aggravate the situation.

Many Common Drugs Affect Weight and Blood Sugar

Many commonly prescribed drugs have the undesirable side effect of altering the metabolism of sugars and fats. In doing so, they increase your likelihood of gaining weight and developing diabetes.

Most prescription medications are inherently dangerous and must be used with extreme care. In one study, researchers calculated that more than 100,000 hospitalized patients die each year from medication errors and more than 2 million others suffer serious side effects. These numbers are shocking because everyone assumes that rigorous controls would be in place in hospitals. Another 700,000 people are hospitalized each year because of adverse reactions to prescription and over-the-counter medications.

Many drugs can lead to weight gain; these include

- Antihistamines (antiallergy, anticold)
- Corticosteroids (immune suppressor, anti-inflammatory)
- Glipizide (insulin releaser)
- Prozac (antidepressant)
- Risperdal (antipsychotic)
- Sulfonylureas (insulin releasers)
- Thiazolidinedione (insulin sensitizer)
- Zoloft (antidepressant)
- Zyprexa (antipsychotic)

Many drugs can reduce glucose tolerance and increase your risk of developing prediabetes and diabetes; these include

- Diazoxide (hypoglycemic)
- Duloxetina (analgesic for diabetic nerve disease)
- Gatifloxacin (antibiotic)
- Oral contraceptives (birth control)
- Thiazides (diuretics)
- Zyprexa (antipsychotic)

Still other drugs interfere with the body's use of vitamins and minerals involved in maintaining normal glucose tolerance. They include

- Antibiotics, which interfere with the B vitamins
- Beta-blockers, which interfere with coenzyme Q10
- Metformin, which interferes with vitamins B6, B12, folic acid, and coenzyme Q10
- Oral contraceptives, which interfere with the B vitamins
- Proton-pump inhibitors, which interfere with vitamins B12 and C
- Thiazides, which interfere with magnesium, potassium, and zinc

Metformin, one of the most commonly prescribed drugs for prediabetes and diabetes, interferes with the body's absorption and use of folic acid (a B vitamin) and vitamin B12. In 2006, researchers reported in the *Archives of Internal Medicine* that people taking either high doses of metformin or taking the drug for more than a couple of years were more than twice as likely to suffer from vitamin B12 deficiency. Low levels of vitamin B12 increase the risk of heart disease, Alzheimer's disease, and cancer.

Some diabetes drugs reduce blood-sugar levels but do not prevent the progression of prediabetes to diabetes. According to a report in the *New England Journal of Medicine*, people taking ramipril (Altace) to treat prediabetes benefited from improved blood-sugar levels; however, the drug did not reduce their risk of developing diabetes or dying.

Early in 2007, Eli Lilly, the maker of Zyprexa (noted previously) agreed to pay a total of $1.2 billion to 28,500 people who took the drug for bipolar disease or schizophrenia. The drug had gained a reputation for promoting both obesity and diabetes.

Likewise, in early 2007, researchers at the Cleveland Clinic published an analysis of forty-two studies involving the antidiabetes drug rosiglitazone (Avandia). They reported that the drug increased the risk of heart attack by 43 percent.

Surviving the Disease-Care System

Serious side effects from drugs are symptomatic of a much greater problem: modern medicine and health care are geared more toward disease diagnosis and management than toward preventing disease.

In 2006, a series of in-depth articles in the *New York Times* described some of the economics of health care that are specific to diabetes. One in eight people in New York City has diabetes, and four hospitals there established programs to help diabetics manage their disease through diet, exercise, and blood-sugar monitoring. The programs were a remarkable success and had a high rate of patient participation, but the hospitals shut down three of the diabetes programs by the time the articles were published. The reason? The hospitals made more money from treating the complications of diabetes than by preventing or controlling the disease. In fact, the hospitals often lost money when it came to prevention.

We all hear about how better nutrition, more exercise, and vitamin supplements could save the United States (and other nations) billions of dollars in health-care costs. So why doesn't the health-care system focus on prevention? The reason is really very simple. If we were to save, let's say, $10 billion in health-care costs, someone else would lose $10 billion in revenues. Junk-food companies, drug makers, surgical instrument companies, hospitals, and physicians would probably be the biggest losers.

The *New York Times* articles pointed out that in the treatment of diabetes, insurers balked at paying $75 for a nutritional consultation, but they were willing to pay more than $300 for each dialysis treatment (due to diabetes-related kidney disease). Likewise, insurers hesitated to pay $150 for a visit to a podiatrist, who can address diabetes-related foot problems, but the insurers would pay more than $30,000 for an amputation.

Even though most hospitals are technically nonprofit corporations, they are very much interested in earning a profit instead of taking a loss. Success in health care is often based on revenues, profits, and large numbers of patients. While stomach-stapling surgery can earn $50,000 for a hospital, there's little financial incentive to pay a nutritionist $100 an hour to provide regular counseling sessions to patients. As the late Emanuel Cheraskin, M.D., D.M.D., once quipped, "Medicine is America's fastest growing failing business."

PART TWO

The Stop Prediabetes Now Program

4

Easy Ways to Curb Your Appetite

Now you understand that one of the main causes of people becoming overweight and prediabetic is eating too many sugary foods, sugarlike carbohydrates, and trans fats. Because rapid increases in blood sugar are followed by steep declines (until people develop full-blown diabetes), individuals quickly become hungry again after eating. Invariably, many opt for the quick pick-me-up of refined sugar and carbs, making blood-sugar levels worse and promoting weight gain.

In this chapter we focus on foods that break this vicious up-and-down blood-sugar cycle, so that you feel less hungry and eat smaller quantities of food. As a general rule, fresh foods improve blood sugar and support weight loss. In contrast, processed and refined foods are usually altered in ways that raise your risk of developing prediabetes and becoming overweight. Some of the specific foods we recommend can improve your blood-sugar levels and curb your appetite within hours, such as between breakfast and lunch! We are not exaggerating—the effect has been demonstrated many times in scientific studies.

Specifically, boosting your consumption of high-quality protein and fiber is central to reducing your blood-sugar levels and appetite. We'll provide you with specific food suggestions here and in other chapters. Several individual foods and condiments also have remarkable benefits on blood sugar, weight, or both. These foods include vinegar, grapefruit, cinnamon, and chili pepper.

Nutrient-Dense Foods and Nutritionally Balanced Eating

Throughout this book we recommend eating a mix of foods that are rich in protein and high in fiber, and we describe our approach as *protein rich*, not high protein. In addition, we'd like you to think of this as an *eating style*, not a diet per se. People tend to go on and off diets, but an eating style is really a long-term habit. It becomes part of your overall lifestyle.

By following our suggestions, you will get the most nutritional value with each calorie or bite of food. Protein-rich foods are *nutrient dense*— that is, they provide a wealth of vitamins and minerals in addition to the protein. Likewise, fiber-rich vegetables and fruits are also nutrient dense. Both protein and fiber help to control your blood sugar and your weight.

Looked at another way, it's foolish to waste calories consuming nutrient-poor soft drinks, juices, candy bars, bread, ice cream, pizza, and pasta. These foods have little to offer nutritionally besides sugar and refined carbs, and they have already compromised your health.

Protein-Rich Foods without Saturated Fat

Over the last few years, medical journals have published dozens of studies that support the benefits of protein in treating prediabetes, overweight, or high blood fats. These studies show that people lose weight and improve their blood sugar when they follow either strict high-protein diets or more moderate diets that substitute a little more protein for a little less carb.

One concern about protein is that it contains large amounts of saturated fat; however, a protein-rich diet does not have to equate with eating a lot of saturated fat. By selecting fish and lean cuts of chicken, turkey, and grass-fed or game meats, it's easy to get sufficient protein while consuming very little saturated fat.

QUICK TIP

What to Do When You Break Your Diet

Nearly all of us occasionally eat foods we shouldn't, such as sweets. The trouble is, once you start it's hard to stop eating those foods. So, how do you get back to your regular eating habits? One way is to eat a lot of protein and no carbs for a day. Doing so helps to stabilize your blood sugar and dampen food cravings. Another way is to brush your teeth several times during the day. Most foods, even those you crave, don't taste very good right after you brush.

Furthermore, by adding plenty of high-fiber, nonstarchy vegetables and fruit—as we recommend—a protein-rich eating plan becomes more nutritionally balanced than traditional high-protein diets. Small amounts of complex carbohydrates can be included, depending on a person's weight and glucose tolerance.

This balanced approach to eating is so obvious that it astounds us that so few people have recommended it. As you read on, you will see that we draw on both common sense and science in encouraging people to eat sensibly.

Why Protein Is Good for You

With the popularity of high-protein, low-carb diets, food companies tried to capitalize by marketing hundreds of low-carb but highly processed foods, from pancake mixes to salad dressings. Most of these processed low-carb foods were not nutritionally sound, and many tasted awful.

Not surprisingly, low-carb processed foods were a flop. When these products failed to sell, the processed food industry argued that the low-carb boom was over, perhaps hoping that people would go back to eating more profitable carbs.

In actuality, interest in high-protein, low-carb foods has not waned. Rather, it continues to evolve into many nutritious variations. Protein is necessary for health and especially for controlling blood sugar, and reducing sugar and other carbs is a sensible way to limit foods that provide only calories and no other nutritional value.

Protein, Blood Sugar, and Weight

Protein is an essential nutrient and, aside from water, serves as the main constituent of our bodies. Some researchers have called it the workhorse of the body because almost every biochemical process depends on protein. Our skin, hair, fingernails, internal organs, and hormones (to name but a few) are all made from protein.

In ancient times, a 150-pound person consumed about 210 grams of protein daily. Today's official governmental recommendation is for just two-fifths that amount. In the past, people obtained about 30 percent of their calories from protein. Today, the official recommendation is for only 12 percent, which is too low for most people. When you don't eat enough protein, it's easy to eat too many sugars and carbs.

What's so good about protein?

- *Protein stabilizes blood sugar.* Protein does not usually increase blood sugar, and in some people, protein can lead to a slight decrease in blood sugar. When blood sugar levels don't go up and down like a roller coaster, people are less likely to have hunger jags and to overeat.

  In a study at the Veterans Administration Medical Center in Minneapolis, Minnesota, researchers placed men on a high-fat, moderately high-protein, and low-carb diet for five weeks. The men's blood-sugar levels decreased by more than a third, and their HbA_{1c} (glycated hemoglobin) levels dropped by 22 percent. The researchers calculated that if the men had stayed on the diet longer, their HbA_{1c} levels would have dropped by half!

- *Protein reduces appetite and creates a "full" feeling.* Protein increases satiety after eating, partly by suppressing the appetite. People have less desire to eat, so protein-rich (low-carb) eating habits quickly turn into low-calorie eating habits. This is particularly good for people who are overly sensitive to carbohydrate calories.

Some research suggests that fish protein is better than meat protein. In one study, Swedish researchers found that eating a pan-fried fish burger for lunch led to an 11 percent reduction in calories consumed at dinner. The subjects felt full with a smaller amount of food, and they did not increase their calorie consumption the next day to make up the difference.

At the University of Washington School of Medicine, Seattle, researchers found that high-protein diets resulted in subjects eating 400 fewer calories daily and a loss of eight pounds over twelve weeks. In this study, the subjects ate the same amount of carbs, but they substituted some of their dietary fat for protein.

- *Protein boosts the metabolic rate.* Your metabolic rate governs how well or how poorly your body burns calories. Studies have consistently found that people lose more fat and less muscle on higher-protein diets. This is important because muscle is the body's principal fat-burning tissue. In a study at the University of Illinois, women on high-protein diets had increases in their thyroid hormone and a faster metabolic rate, which helped them to burn calories. Protein also requires a fair amount of energy to metabolize, resulting in a thermogenic effect three times higher than that of either carbohydrate or fat.

- *Protein plus exercise burns even more fat.* Researchers at the University of Illinois, Urbana, placed obese middle-age women on either a high-protein, low-carb diet or a high-carb, low-protein diet. They also asked some of the women to exercise regularly. All of the subjects lost weight, but those following the high-protein diet, and those on the high-protein diet who exercised lost the most body fat and the least muscle. The combination of a high-protein diet and exercise led to a 21.4 percent reduction in body fat. In contrast, women on the high-carbohydrate diet who didn't exercise lost only 12.8 percent of their body fat.

- *Protein helps to preserve muscle.* Protein helps you to maintain muscle, the best tissue for burning sugar, carbs, and fats. In contrast, simple low-calorie diets lead to a significant loss of muscle. Some of the protein you eat is used to make and maintain muscle, the tissue that most efficiently burns fat. Preserving your muscle mass becomes especially important after age forty, when age-related muscle loss accelerates. Physical activity also helps to make and maintain muscle.

- *Protein does not increase the risk of developing heart disease.* In a major study, researchers at Harvard University found that high-protein, low-carb diets did *not* increase the risk of developing heart disease, compared with diets containing large amounts of carbohydrates. When the subjects included a fair amount of vegetable protein in their diets, their risk of developing heart disease actually went down. Still other research has shown that high-protein diets do not increase cholesterol or blood pressure. As we've explained, it's important to combine lean protein with a lot of vegetables for maximum health benefits.

The bottom line is that protein is good for you. When you increase the amount of high-quality protein you eat, you do a better job of regulating your blood sugar and weight.

Glucagon, the Hormone behind Protein's Benefits

One fundamental reason why protein is beneficial relates to its glucagon-boosting effect. This hormone counteracts insulin, and most of what it does is in direct opposition to insulin. Of course, we need both hormones for health, and they tend to interact like the ends of a seesaw.

For example, while insulin helps to convert blood sugar to fat, glucagon blocks this conversion. Whereas insulin helps us to store fat, glucagon helps to burn it. The key is striking a balance in a world where most processed and refined foods increase insulin and suppress glucagon.

Glucagon has many other beneficial actions. It raises blood-sugar levels when you are experiencing low blood sugar. In fact, the fastest and best way to stabilize your blood sugar is to eat a little protein.

CATHERINE'S STORY
Reversing Diabetes with Diet and Supplements

In her late sixties, Catherine was a widow and a retired teacher. Friends told Catherine that her weight was fine, but she had felt for years that she was a little overweight. Her blood pressure was elevated (140/86 mmHg), but the real shock came when her regular physician diagnosed her with diabetes. Routine blood tests found Catherine's fasting blood sugar up to 124 mg/dl and her triglycerides at 200 mg/dl.

She felt devastated by the news. Catherine clearly understood the health consequences of diabetes because her aunt has the disease.

Motivated, she moved quickly to turn her life around. She learned how to cook and eat protein-rich, low-carb foods and completely cleaned out all of her cookie stashes and bread bins. Catherine also made an appointment with Dr. Ron at the Center for the Improvement of Human Functioning International, where they jointly reviewed all of her supplements. She increased her omega-3 supplements (which help to lower triglycerides) and added chromium and alpha-lipoic acid (which improve insulin function and lower blood sugar).

Two months later, Catherine had lost ten pounds. At a follow-up visit, she mentioned feeling much better physically and clearer mentally, although she thought she had felt all right before. Her fasting blood sugar was now 85 mg/dl, and her triglycerides were 110 mg/dl. Her blood pressure had also decreased to 120/75 mmHg. Now she definitely was not diabetic.

Catherine's improvements occurred so quickly that she started to wonder whether her original doctor's diagnosis of diabetes was even correct. Nonetheless, she was delighted that she felt so much better, and she made it clear that she would continue to improve her health.

QUICK TIP

Protein for Vegetarians

People often ask us about adapting our recommendations for vegetarians. Eggs, fish, hard cheeses, and yogurt can substitute for meat and fowl. If you do not eat fish, dairy products, or eggs, it becomes much more difficult to follow our eating plan. While legumes are considered a good source of protein, they also contain fairly large amounts of carbs.

If you are a vegetarian who is prediabetic or overweight, you must consider whether your current eating habits have contributed to your health problems. If that's the case, a vegetarian diet may not be suited to you. Sometimes vegetarians eat far too many carbs in the form of bread, pasta, fruit juices, and sweets—and not enough vegetables.

You could consider glucagon the body's energy hormone, in contrast to insulin, which is the fat-storage hormone. Glucagon stimulates the release of stored sugar, called glycogen, and its conversion into glucose. (Most people have about sixty to ninety minutes' worth of liver glycogen, which can be used up in strenuous exercise.)

Glucagon also promotes the breakdown of both fat and protein for energy. In addition, glucagon lowers cholesterol production, which insulin increases. It's also a mild diuretic, signaling the kidneys to release water from the body and combating water weight.

Why Fiber Is Good for You

High-protein diets have frequently been criticized for their lack of vegetables and fruits. Our protein-rich eating plan corrects this problem by recommending that you eat high-fiber, nonstarchy vegetables and fruits. Fiber reduces blood-sugar and insulin levels, and people who eat more fiber are generally thinner than those who don't. High-fiber fruits and vegetables also contain lots of vitamins, minerals, and other nutrients.

In ancient times, the average person ate 104 grams of fiber daily. Fiber was consumed in many types of plant foods, including greens, root vegetables, fruits, nuts, and seeds. Today, official government recommendations call for 20 to 30 grams of fiber daily, but most Americans get only

10 to 20 grams. They're constipated, bloated, and at risk of developing high blood-sugar levels.

Fiber Helps You to Manage Your Blood Sugar and Weight

The fiber in vegetables and fruits plays a central role in regulating blood sugar and weight. Most high-fiber foods are also very low in starch and low on the glycemic index. Although they contain some naturally occurring sugars and starches, the fiber slows their digestion and thereby moderates their effect on blood-sugar levels. Increasing your fiber intake—in foods, not supplements—will lower your blood-sugar levels and help you to lose weight.

Although fiber is not digested, it helps to move food through the digestive tract, thereby promoting regular bowel movements and leaving you feeling less stuffed and constipated. Everyone knows what relief a good bowel movement brings! Long term, fiber reduces the chances of developing diverticulosis and diverticulitis, two intestinal diseases caused by eating too many highly processed foods. Along the way, fiber helps to create beneficial compounds that activate cancer-protecting genes.

Vegetables and fruits contain three types of fiber. One, insoluble fiber, sometimes called roughage, helps to move food through the lower digestive tract. The second type, soluble fiber, absorbs water and forms

---

QUICK TIP

Chew Your Food Well

To get the maximum amount of nutrients from your food, chew it well. This means chewing for about ten seconds per bite, not chewing a couple of times and then swallowing. The more you chew, the smaller the food particles become, and the more they get coated with carbohydrate- and protein-digesting enzymes in the mouth. That's the first step in digestion, and the efficiency of later steps in your stomach and intestines depends on the first step. Besides, chewing your food gives you time to enjoy the taste and the texture of what you eat. Don't rush it—savor your food.

a gel-like mass, which stabilizes blood sugar. The third, fermentable fiber, is good for the gut bacteria that help you to digest food. Fermentable fiber includes pectin, found in berries and apples, and inulin (no relation to insulin), found in avocados.

Some scientific research studies have found that fiber can lower post-meal levels of blood sugar and insulin in both overweight and normal-weight subjects. People with diabetes who boost their fiber to 50 grams daily can lower their blood-sugar levels by 10 percent and, in the long term, can reduce their risk of developing diabetes and becoming overweight.

With few exceptions, we usually recommend that you get fiber from nonstarchy vegetables and fruits, such as dark lettuces, tomatoes, cucumbers, avocado, spinach, broccoli, cauliflower, asparagus, mushrooms, radishes, bell peppers, snow peas (with edible pods), zucchini squash, mustard greens, endive, collard greens, and chicory. Nonstarchy fruits include raspberries, blueberries, blackberries, strawberries, apples, kiwifruit, and pomegranate seeds. Potatoes, bananas, oranges, and pears are especially high in sugars and other rapidly digested starches, so avoid them until your blood sugar and weight improve.

Why Grains Aren't That Great

Whole-wheat and multigrain breads are often promoted as a good source of fiber and other nutrients, but all grains are heavily processed, resulting in smaller, more rapidly absorbed particles of starch. Whole-grain foods are promoted as being nutritious, but whatever nutrients they provide come in greater amounts in protein and vegetables. Whole grains have far less nutrient density than lean protein and vegetables.

We have other concerns with breads, pastas, cereals, and other grain-based foods—what scientists call cereal grains. About one in every hundred people has celiac disease, a severe intolerance of gluten that can lead to malabsorption and nutritional deficiencies. Gluten is a protein found in wheat, rye, and barley products and sometimes in oats. Some evidence suggests that half of all people may be sensitive to gluten.

If you are gluten tolerant and your weight and blood sugar are normal, you can occasionally indulge in one of several grain products. Low-carb whole-wheat tortillas contain about 4 grams of carbs per tortilla.

European-style black breads, with obvious seeds and husks, have a bit more in the way of carbs, but they also have considerably larger fiber particles. Buckwheat is not a grain and, aside from its calories or carbs, should not cause grain-related problems.

Other Foods That Help Your Blood Sugar and Weight

Years ago, fad diets recommended vinegar and grapefruit to help people lose weight. At the time, there wasn't any scientific evidence that they worked. Now there's credible research showing that vinegar, grapefruit, and a few other foods can improve blood sugar, insulin, and weight.

Vinegar

People with impaired glucose tolerance often crave foods made with vinegar, such as dill pickles, certain types of gravies, and vinaigrette salad dressings. It's almost as if their bodies are begging for foods to help regulate their blood-sugar levels.

Vinegar has been used medicinally for at least two thousand years. Its pungency comes from acetic acid, which inhibits the activity of carbohydrate-digesting enzymes, including amylase, sucrase, lactase, and maltase. When these enzymes are blocked, sugar and starches pass through the digestive tract much the same way that indigestible fiber does. You could consider vinegar a natural and inexpensive starch blocker. Any type of vinegar has this effect—white vinegar, balsamic vinegar, apple-cider vinegar, and red-wine vinegar—as long as it contains at least 5 percent acetic acid.

> **A Point to Remember**
>
> Use vinegar liberally in salad dressings and in other dishes. It helps to regulate blood sugar and suppress appetite.

Acetic acid also helps to convert glucose to glycogen, your muscle's reserve fuel. This is good, and it helps athletes during their postexercise recovery. Another advantage is that increased conversion of glucose to glycogen reduces insulin requirements. These mechanisms are similar to how the diabetes drugs acarbose and metformin work to decrease blood sugar, but vinegar is cheaper and safer than those medications.

Vinegar, blood sugar, and insulin. Recent research by separate teams of U.S. and Swedish researchers has given vinegar new scientific credibility. In 2004, Carol S. Johnston, Ph.D., a nutrition professor and researcher at Arizona State University, Mesa, reported that consuming a small amount of apple-cider vinegar significantly diminishes postmeal increases in glucose and insulin. Such a decrease would lessen a person's tendency toward having prediabetes and hunger pangs. Johnston found that after prediabetic people consumed a little vinegar, their insulin function improved by 34 percent; the insulin function in those with diabetes improved almost 20 percent. Even the healthy subjects had a better response to the carbs.

Swedish scientists saw similar benefits. Postmeal increases in blood sugar decreased by 43 percent, and postmeal increases in insulin decreased by 31 percent. Subjects also felt less hungry thirty minutes, ninety minutes, and two hours after eating.

Vinegar and weight loss. In follow-up studies, Johnston investigated whether vinegar might lower cholesterol levels. It didn't—but it did, unexpectedly, help people to lose weight. She asked thirty people to take 2 tablespoons of vinegar or cranberry juice (as a placebo) before lunch and dinner each day for four weeks. People taking the vinegar lost an average of two pounds, and some lost four to five pounds, while those in the placebo group maintained the same weight. Because the study was conducted in November and December, when people commonly eat more than usual, the weight-loss benefits of vinegar may be even greater.

To put this research into practice, make your own vinaigrette dressing for salads. We have some recipes in chapter 8.

Grapefruit Promotes Weight Loss

Since the Hollywood Diet of the 1930s, grapefruit has been included in a variety of weight-loss programs. A recent study found that grapefruit, grapefruit juice, and grapefruit capsules actually helped people to lose weight and improve their insulin function.

Researchers at the Scripps Clinic in San Diego, California, asked ninety-one overweight patients to slightly modify their regular eating habits for twelve weeks. The subjects were asked to eat one-half of a

> ### QUICK TIP
>
> **Avoid Eating Late Dinners**
>
> It's all too easy to work late and then eat a big late dinner, but that's bad news in terms of your blood sugar. First, the stress of working late prompts your body to secrete insulin and cortisol, the two hormones involved in storing fat around your belly. Second, a late dinner means you've delayed eating—in effect, skipped a meal. It's all right to eat a light snack instead of dinner, but a full dinner past 9 p.m. will raise your blood sugar and keep it high by the time you wake up. That will make you feel tired in the morning and will tempt you to skip breakfast (because you're not hungry) and eat more calories during the rest of the day.

fresh grapefruit, drink 8 ounces of grapefruit juice, take grapefruit capsules (containing 500 mg of whole grapefruit), or take placebos three times daily before each meal. People taking capsules were given a small amount of apple juice to match the calories of the grapefruit and the grapefruit juice. In every other respect, the subjects were encouraged to follow their usual eating habits.

By the end of the study, people eating the fresh grapefruit lost an average of 3.6 pounds, those drinking grapefruit juice lost 3.3 pounds, and those taking grapefruit capsules lost 2.4 pounds. In contrast, subjects taking the placebos lost only one-half pound. One-third of the subjects were prediabetic, and those who consumed the fresh juice or the grapefruit benefited from significant reductions in fasting and postmeal insulin levels.

Why would grapefruit have these effects, despite the calories it adds? First, as we discussed in chapter 3, not all calories are equal. Second, grapefruit contains compounds that are known to reduce the activity of the liver enzymes involved in breaking down drugs. It is very possible that grapefruit affects some of the enzymes that help to regulate blood sugar and weight.

Peanuts Help to Control Blood Sugar

Small amounts of peanuts have virtually no impact on blood-sugar levels—and they may reduce postmeal increases in blood sugar.

In another experiment, Carol S. Johnston, Ph.D., fed eleven healthy people meals that were high in either sugar and carbs or protein. For some of the meals, 25 grams of peanut butter or roasted peanuts (about 1 ounce) were substituted for butter. When the peanuts were added to the high-sugar, high-carb meal, the postmeal rise in blood sugar was cut in half.

Chili Lowers Insulin Levels

Foods made with chili are well known for their ability to dilate blood vessels and make people sweat. Chili may have some mild thermogenic, or fat-burning, properties. Researchers recently reported that eating chili-containing meals led to a significant reduction on the postmeal increase in insulin secretion.

The researchers prepared meals with 33 mg of capsaicin (the active ingredient in chili) in roughly a 1-ounce blend of chili. The meals were fed to thirty-six middle-age men and women three times daily for four weeks. Postmeal rises in insulin were one-third lower after people ate the chili-containing meals, compared with otherwise identical bland meals, suggesting improvements in glucose tolerance. The benefits were even greater among overweight subjects.

Although chili can reduce insulin levels, the most common source of chili is in high-carbohydrate and high-dairy Mexican foods. Dairy products result in a low-glycemic response but provoke a very high

---

QUICK TIP

Appetite Control in a Pill?

We're generally skeptical about supplements that claim to suppress appetite, promote weight loss, and block the absorption of starches and fat; however, considerable research shows that several supplements, available at health food stores and pharmacies, can help to reduce appetite. They work in large part by improving blood-sugar levels, and when blood-sugar levels stabilize, so does appetite. These supplements include alpha-lipoic acid and R-lipoic acid, chromium, Super CitriMax, American ginseng, Phase 2 starch neutralizer, and glycine. For more information on these and other supplements, turn to chapter 10.

insulin response, which likely results from responses to the hormones found in dairy products. (After all, dairy products come from hormonally active lactating cows.) Eating chili with low-carbohydrate and low-saturated-fat foods might be preferable. You can, as an example, add chili flakes to vinaigrette salad dressings and to ground meat patties.

Cinnamon Lowers Blood Sugar and Cholesterol

People usually enjoy the taste of cinnamon when it's added to apple cider or baked goods. Putting a small amount of cinnamon in foods or taking cinnamon in capsules can significantly improve blood-sugar levels. Be warned, though: eating a Cinnabon, which has 144 grams of sugars and carbs and 730 calories, won't do anything good for you.

Researchers at the U.S. Department of Agriculture and their counterparts from Pakistan tested the effects of cinnamon-containing capsules on 60 people with diabetes. The subjects' fasting blood-sugar levels ranged from 140 to 400 mg/dl at the beginning of the study. They were asked to take 1, 3, or 6 grams of cinnamon daily after meals, and others were asked to take the same number of capsules containing placebos for forty days. One gram of cinnamon is about one-quarter teaspoon of the ground herb.

Fasting blood-sugar levels decreased by 18 to 29 percent among people taking cinnamon. In addition, cholesterol levels declined by 7 to 27 percent, and triglyceride levels went down 23 to 30 percent. No improvement occurred among people taking the placebos.

You can sprinkle cinnamon powder on fresh fruit, such as strawberries, raspberries, blueberries, pomegranate seeds, and cantaloupe. Ground cinnamon spice is much less expensive than capsules.

In this chapter, we've offered ways to jump-start your recovery from being prediabetic and overweight, mostly by focusing on foods to help control your appetite. In the next chapter, we provide guidelines for improving your overall relationship with food. Later in the book, we'll teach you how to navigate grocery stores, health food markets, specialty markets, and a variety of restaurants.

5

Improve Your Relationship with Food

Prediabetes and overweight are nutritional disorders. Having these health problems is a little like being in a bad relationship: you desire something that you know is wrong for you. If you want to reverse prediabetes and lose weight, you have to develop a healthier relationship with your food.

The key to reversing prediabetes and weight problems is simple in concept: cut back on the number of empty calories (mostly processed sugar and carbs) that you eat and drink, while increasing the amount of nutrient-dense foods that you consume. By following this approach, you'll get more "bang" for your nutritional "buck."

Eating habits can be especially difficult to change. They are shaped by our culture, our upbringing, peer pressure, our education, stress, our income, and the amount of time we have available to plan meals and cook. Many emotions are associated with eating, such as comfort and love.

We don't expect you to make major dietary changes overnight, but we do ask you to work steadily to improve the eating habits that have made you sick. Sometimes this means fighting your craving for french fries and resisting the urge to have dessert. If you have the will, there is a way—and the process may be easier than you think.

As you follow our dietary recommendations, you'll feel better within days and may very well notice an improvement on the first day. Long term, your risk of developing serious diseases will decrease, a change that will be reflected in healthier numbers when you get blood tests at the doctor's office. You can commit to one dietary change today and adopt one or two others each week. Feeling good, avoiding drugs and their side effects, and sidestepping the surgeon's scalpel are among the payoffs.

In this chapter, we'll help you to create a new and lasting foundation for healthy eating, built around three themes:

1. Five essential daily habits to follow wherever you are,

2. Six principles that define your new relationship with food, and

3. Ten practical guidelines that will steer you toward your specific eating habits and food choices.

Are you starting to wonder how much work this will take? You have a choice: to keep doing what has made you sick and will shorten your life, or to do what will make you healthier and will lengthen your life.

Five Essential Daily Habits

We recommend that you follow our five essential daily habits every single day. They'll get you off to a good start each morning and keep you going through the day.

Essential Daily Habit #1. Eat Breakfast

We grew up hearing that breakfast was the most important meal of the day. The more we learn, the more we realize how true this is—and the type of breakfast is of paramount importance.

Breakfast literally means to break your fast of the previous ten to twelve hours (most of which you've slept through). Skipping breakfast creates prediabetic changes in insulin function and also raises total cholesterol and "bad" low-density lipoprotein cholesterol. Having just coffee, juice, and a bagel, or a bowl of a sugary cereal, isn't any better.

To improve your blood-sugar levels, curb your appetite, and lose weight, it's essential that you eat a protein-rich breakfast each and every morning. People who eat a couple of eggs for breakfast are less hungry for the rest of the day and for much of the following day. Because they're less hungry, they also eat less. In one study, scientists reported that an egg-and-toast breakfast led to people eating 420 fewer calories over the following day and a half.

If you don't like eggs, you can eat a few bites of leftover chicken or another high-protein food, along with a small amount of fresh fruit. You can get somewhat similar benefits by eating a low-glycemic sugar-free cereal, such as oatmeal (so long as it is not instant oatmeal and does not contain any sugars). Still, our first choice would be eggs.

Essential Daily Habit #2. Eat at Regular Times

Pressures at work and home, and being short of time in general, can sabotage your best intentions to eat well. When you feel stressed, your good eating habits are usually the first thing to slide—you delay or skip meals, or succumb to sweets and fast foods. That's when your blood sugar sinks, then rockets too high, and then sinks again. (You can read more about stress and eating habits in Jack's previous book *The Food-Mood Solution*.)

Because of life's pressures, you need to be especially vigilant about eating at regular times. Grant yourself this time, just as you would if you had to go to the toilet. Food provides the fuel for your brain and your body, and when you don't eat, you don't function at your best.

You can brown bag your lunch and reheat tasty leftovers from our recipes. Alternatively, you can go to a nearby supermarket and get some sliced deli turkey and cheese and an apple, or cooked shrimp and sugar-free cocktail sauce or salsa.

If you often face busy, lunch-crunching days, stash some food in your office (or in a cooler in your car or truck, if you're out on calls). You can make a roll-up with a low-carb whole-wheat tortilla stuffed with just about any kind of meat and cheese. You can also make your own trail mix and keep that handy—although it's not a meal, it'll keep you going for an extra hour or so. (See more under "Choose Your Snacks Carefully.")

Reversing Prediabetes and Weight Problems

The onset of menopause had not been kind to Liz. At five foot, four inches tall and 150 pounds, she was overweight. Five years ago, when Liz was fifty-five, her hot flashes, vaginal dryness, and low bone density were compounded by the diagnosis of uncontrolled hypertension. Her family physician started her on hormone-replacement therapy and blood pressure medication.

Lab tests foretold future problems: elevated cholesterol and triglycerides, and a prediabetic glucose level of 111 mg/dl. Tests also found her to have low levels of magnesium, a mineral involved in glucose and cholesterol metabolism.

Liz started to take some supplements, including magnesium and calcium, and also began to walk two miles each day. She soon lost ten pounds but then inexplicably started to gain weight. Each year, she added about another five pounds, and her blood pressure crept up even higher. Her family doctor prescribed various blood pressure medications.

Liz's turning point came after she underwent preventive medical tests at the Center for the Improvement of Human Functioning. Her blood fats were still elevated: her total cholesterol was 257 mg/dl, her triglycerides were 209 mg/dl, her "bad" low-density lipoprotein cholesterol was 169 mg/dl, and her "good" high-density lipoprotein was a relatively low 46. Liz's HbA_{1c} (a snapshot of recent blood-sugar levels) was 6.5%, well above normal. Her C-reactive protein (CRP), a marker of inflammation and heart disease risk, was almost three times higher than normal. Her prediabetes was progressing toward true diabetes.

Liz's sister, brother, and grandfather had already been diagnosed with diabetes, and they suffered from some of the disease's complications: nerve damage, hypertension, heart failure, and stroke. Many of these complications stem from chronic low-grade inflammation, and Liz's elevated CRP level confirmed the link. She, too, would develop diabetic complications if nothing changed, and that fact turned out to be her motivator.

Liz was determined not to suffer the same medical fate as her family members. She greatly reduced her intake of sweets and breads, while eating smaller meals, more vegetables, and a couple of healthy snacks each day. She took a janitorial job to be more physically active, in addition to her daily two-mile walk.

Dr. Ron asked her to take alpha-lipoic acid (300 mg twice daily), biotin (10 mg daily), and an extract of red yeast rice (600 mg twice daily, to help lower blood fats). Liz was determined and, by sticking to her plan, she lost twenty-one pounds in the first three months and another ten pounds four months later.

Her numbers improved significantly: her cholesterol was down to 142 mg/dl, her triglycerides to 66 mg/dl, and her LDL to 86 mg/dl. These are all impressive changes for someone to achieve without resorting to drugs. Although Liz's HDL remained about the same at 43 mg/dl, the ratio between HDL and other blood fats improved significantly, another good sign. And that wasn't all. Her HbA_{1c} dropped down to 5.8, which was almost normal, and her fasting blood sugar decreased to 102 mg/dl.

Liz's prediabetes was better but not entirely gone. She understood that she could no longer take her health for granted and that she had to work to improve it. She was able to stop taking one of her blood pressure medications, and she felt much better than she had in years.

Essential Daily Habit #3. Eat Slowly and Enjoy Your Food

Time pressures and the anxieties they generate force people to eat quickly, and one of every four Americans ends up at a fast-food restaurant each day of the week. The fast-food industry is based on the idea of food that's quick to serve and quick to eat. But the faster people eat, the more they eat. So to eat less, it helps to eat slower.

Kathleen J. Melanson, Ph.D., of the University of Rhode Island, Kingston, studied the eating habits of thirty young women in a laboratory setting. On one day, she asked the women to eat a meal as quickly as possible without pausing. On another day, she asked them to take small bites and chew each bite fifteen to twenty times.

When the women ate fast, they consumed an average of 646 calories in just nine minutes. When they took their time, they ate only 579 calories in twenty-nine minutes, an 11 percent difference. Eating slowly also left the women feeling more satisfied right after eating, as well as an hour later.

It's far more satisfying, and less stressful, to take the time to enjoy your food.

Essential Daily Habit #4. Eat Smaller Portions

According to the Hartman Group, which conducts market research for food and supplement companies, most people understand the importance of controlling food-portion sizes, but they find the practicalities difficult and exasperating. That's not surprising. Portion sizes can be vague, confusing, and misleading. For example, a study published in the *Annals of Internal Medicine* reported that people accurately estimated calories in small meals but underestimated the number of calories in large meals by almost 40 percent.

Without clear indicators, it's not easy to figure out reasonable portion sizes. The number of servings (portions) listed in the Nutrition Facts boxes of packaged foods is practically meaningless, and many food companies understate serving sizes so that people think foods are low in sugar, carbs, or fats. But unrealistically small servings leave people unsatisfied, so they end up eating more.

What's a modest serving? A serving of protein or vegetables is roughly the size of the palm of your hand or a deck of cards. A serving of starchy foods would be a little smaller. You can certainly eat larger quantities of vegetables and salads, and their bulk will help to fill you up.

None of this means you're forever prohibited from eating a second helping, but you probably should avoid doing so as a regular habit. Eat your meal and wait five to ten minutes before deciding whether to have seconds.

If you're eating in a restaurant, and the food covers all or most of your plate, mentally divide (or literally divide with your knife) what you will eat and what you're going to take home. Alternatively, you can split an entrée with a friend, order a smaller entrée, or get just a couple of appetizers, or tapas.

Essential Daily Habit #5. Choose Your Snacks Carefully

Years ago, snacks were considered special treats, such as the occasional cookie and glass of milk after school. Somehow, snacking has morphed into all-day grazing. According to the Hartman Group, people now snack throughout the day, either impulsively eating (because the idea pops into their head) or compulsively eating (because they can't stop).

Because of frequent up-and-down blood-sugar swings, people frequently get hungry and snack between meals, while others routinely eat snacks instead of lunch. They also snack in front of the television, at sports games, at their desks, and in their cars. Snacking displaces more nutritious foods because snackers aren't always hungry enough for a more nutritious lunch or dinner.

Some people feel that they eat less through snacking, when in fact they eat more. They can also be very protective of their snacks, guarding them with the emotional attachment of an addiction.

As blood sugar improves, the temptation to snack decreases. That's because you will be less hungry between meals. Still, because of work pressures, you may occasionally have little choice but to snack. At times like this, a little snack planning (instead of a snack attack) can keep your overall eating habits on track.

Nuts and seeds make for a high-quality snack. They provide a mix of protein, carbs, fiber, and fats, and some research has shown that eating just two ounces of nuts daily can reduce postmeal increases in blood sugar and insulin. Because of the carbs in nuts, however, it's important to limit the quantity you eat. To avoid overeating nuts, don't snack on them straight out of a bag or a can. Instead, transfer a measured amount of the nuts to a small plate. (See our Trail Mix recipe on page 189.)

Food-Philosophy Principles for Positive Eating Habits

These six principles form the tenets of good eating habits. We call them philosophical principles because they are higher level, more general guidelines.

Food-Philosophy Principle #1. Be Mindful of What You Eat

People frequently stuff almost anything into their mouths without giving it much thought. They drive through McDonald's without considering other meal options, and they are oblivious to the enormous quantities of calories and carbs in a burger, fries, and a soft drink.

Being mindful means paying attention, thinking before you eat—in this case, before you put food or drink in your mouth. If you're a mindful shopper, you examine the list of ingredients on food packages and reject unhealthy foods. When you're mindful, you're less likely to have that unnecessary second helping or to snack out of boredom. You're also more likely to savor and enjoy your food, relishing each bite.

Food-Philosophy Principle #2. Eat a Diversity of Foods

People often get into a rut when it comes to their eating habits. For example, most people who do eat vegetables tend to eat the same narrow range of vegetables, such as potatoes, peas, carrots, and corn.

A diversity of foods provides a variety of nutrients. It also offers a tantalizing panoply of tastes and flavors that you would otherwise miss. A salad with romaine or Bibb lettuce provides more vitamins, minerals, and vitaminlike nutrients than, say, a salad with low-nutrition iceberg lettuce. Tossing in some spinach leaves, endive, arugula, or watercress adds different nutrients and flavors to your meal and cuts down on the boredom factor.

Food-Philosophy Principle #3. Opt for Fresh Foods

There's almost always a huge difference in nutritional quality between fresh foods and those that come in boxes, cans, jars, bottles, and bags.

Fresh foods are usually less expensive because they have undergone less processing. They may take a little more time to prepare but not that much more—and we give you recipes and preparation shortcuts in chapter 8.

Fresh foods typically resemble what they looked like in nature—a sign of minimal processing and handling. Most foods sold in boxes, cans, jars, bottles, and bags have added sugar, refined sugarlike carbs, or trans fats. Canned foods tend to have a higher glycemic index—more of a sugar-like effect—because sitting in water breaks down much of their fiber. Frozen foods are acceptable when fresh ones aren't available, but read the Ingredients list carefully, and reject foods with unhealthy ingredients.

Food-Philosophy Principle #4. Don't Take Food for Granted

Over the last hundred years, many nations have made great strides in sanitation and hygiene, resulting in a food supply that is mostly free of disease-causing bacteria. We believe that the near elimination of bacterially contaminated food has led to a sense of complacency: if food is clean and free of germs that make us sick, it should be good to eat, right?

Fast-food restaurants, such as McDonald's and Burger King, follow stringent rules to avoid bacterial contamination of food. You're not likely to get food poisoning at these and other fast-food restaurants. But this doesn't mean most fast foods are healthy. Don't assume that fast foods are safe to eat because they're prepared in clean kitchens. Germ-free or not, fast foods contribute in a big way to prediabetes and over-weight.

Food-Philosophy Principle #5. Don't Assume Anything about the Food You Buy

Jack once bought a bag of dried cranberries, thinking they would be a nice addition to a salad. After all, cranberries are loaded with vitamins and minerals. But on this occasion, Jack neglected to read the list of ingredients. Cranberries are tart, and these dried cranberries contained added sugar to make them sweeter.

The Latin phrase *caveat emptor* means "Let the buyer beware." You alone are responsible for what you buy and eat. You wouldn't buy a television or a car without reading at least some of the fine print and learning about the warranty. Don't buy any packaged foods (in boxes, cans, jars, bottles, or bags) without reading the fine print on the side or the back of the package. Reject any food with unhealthy or unnecessary ingredients. We explain how to read food labels in chapter 6.

Food-Philosophy Principle #6. Eat Organic Food as Often as You Can Afford It

Organic foods are grown without pesticides and with farming methods that sustain soil quality. You can buy organic vegetables, fruits, dairy products, and eggs at natural food stores, specialty markets (such as Trader Joe's), and many supermarkets. You can even get a few organic foods at Costco and Wal-Mart.

Organic produce has higher nutrient levels for a number of reasons. One, organic farming is usually a low-yield operation compared with high-yield commercial farming. Research by Donald R. Davis, Ph.D., of the University of Texas, Austin, has shown that an acre of soil has only so much nutrition to give. High-yield farming dilutes that nutrition among a larger number of plants. Two, pesticides reduce plants' production of vitamins and other antioxidants.

When you can, buy grass- or range-fed meat or fowl, although they may not be organic per se. Animals that graze on grass have a healthy fat profile—high in the omega-3 fats—similar to that of wild salmon. The omega-3s support more natural insulin function and promote weight loss, compared with saturated fats and omega-6 fats. That said, grass-fed, range-fed, and game meats tend to be much leaner and therefore may be better cooked medium rare, slow-cooked (braised or in a crock pot), made into burgers, or marinated. Corn-fed beef has more saturated fat and a less healthy fat profile in general.

With fish, select wild instead of farmed whenever possible. Packages of fresh fish are usually labeled as to their origin; if they're not, the clerk at the fish counter should know. Wild fish come mostly from the oceans, although some may be caught in lakes or rivers. Farmed fish are fed grains, just like corn-fed cows. They tend to have a higher percentage of undesirable omega-6 fats and more pesticides and chemical contaminants.

Practical Guidelines for
Healthy Eating Habits

Our practical guidelines focus mostly on selecting specific healthy foods and ingredients and avoiding others. These dietary recommendations are essentially our version of the Mediterranean diet. We emphasize high-quality protein such as chicken and fish and a lot of high-fiber vegetables and fruits, olive and macadamia nut oils, and vinegar, but much less starch than in the traditional Mediterranean diet.

You will be able to find many healthy equivalents in natural food stores such as Whole Foods, Wild Oats, and Vitamin Cottage. For example, most commercial brands of mayonnaise, such as Kraft, use soybean oil, which is not as healthy as other oils. Most natural food stores carry Spectrum Naturals Canola Mayonnaise, which uses naturally processed canola oil, pasteurized eggs, honey, and other natural ingredients. Peanut butter is another example. Many supermarket brands use partially hydrogenated vegetable oils to create a smooth texture, while the brands sold in natural food stores typically contain only peanut butter.

Practical Guideline #1. Eat Nutrient-Dense Foods to Make Every Bite Count

Eating healthier foods is about quality over quantity. Nutritious foods are nutrient-dense foods. They're packed with good nutrition in every bite and every calorie—protein, fiber, vitamins, minerals, healthy fats, and other important nutrients. In our opinion, the most nutrient-dense foods are fish, chicken, lean meats, and vegetables.

In contrast, nutrient-poor foods contain mostly sugars and sugarlike carbohydrates that provide few, if any, other nutrients. If you're interested in being healthy, it shouldn't be difficult to choose between nutrient-dense and nutrient-poor foods. A fast-food burger and fries, pizza, a rice bowl, or a burrito fill you up, but they don't give you a lot of nutritional value for your money. They're mostly refined sugar, other carbs, and unhealthy fats.

Practical tip: When deciding what to eat, emphasize mostly protein and vegetables. Eggs for breakfast, a Caesar salad (minus croutons) for lunch, and pan-fried unbreaded fish and vegetables for dinner are all good choices.

Practical Guideline #2. Eat Some High-Quality Protein at Every Meal

High-quality protein is good for your blood sugar. If your blood sugar is elevated, eating protein will help to control it. If your blood sugar swings wildly up and down, protein will help to stabilize it. In the process, protein reduces your appetite. Protein is one of our top nutrient-dense foods.

We're not talking about a super-high Atkins-style protein diet, just a moderate amount of protein forming the core of your breakfast, lunch, and dinner. Fish, chicken, turkey, eggs, and lean cuts of beef, pork, and lamb are all great protein sources. Always trim or drain off excess fat.

Practical tip: Don't dredge your protein (such as fish or chicken) in flour (although a light coating of rice flour is occasionally acceptable) and never deep fry it. Pan-frying is fine as long as you use olive or macadamia nut oil. Try not to overcook your protein because doing so alters its structure and reduces its nutritional value. Roughly 30 to 50 percent of the food on your plate should be protein. Vegetables contain a small amount of protein.

Practical Guideline #3. Eat Plenty of Vegetables

Vegetables are a treasure trove of vitamins, minerals, other nutrients, and fiber, and people who eat the most vegetables have the lowest long-term risk of developing most types of disease. Nonstarchy, high-fiber veggies are best because they have high nutrient density and relatively few carbohydrates. The fiber in veggies buffers your body's response to any naturally occurring sugar.

Unfortunately, the vast majority of Americans (69 to 91 percent, depending on the study) do *not* eat the five recommended daily servings. You'll probably have to make a conscious effort to eat more vegetables. In general, vegetables have more nutritional value and fiber than do fruits.

Practical tip: High-fiber nonstarchy vegetables include salad greens, tomatoes, cucumbers, spinach, broccoli, cauliflower, carrots, and green beans. Avoid all forms of potatoes. Limit your consumption of corn and peas, but snow peas (which are steamed or pan-fried in the pod) are fine.

KIM'S STORY
Her Weight Was Normal, but She Was Preobese

About one in four thin people have elevated insulin levels and insulin resistance, key signs of prediabetes. Kim was one of them.

She was thirty years old, attractive, and slender. But Kim was also flabby and a little self-conscious about how her buttocks (which were not large) jiggled when she wore a bikini and walked on the beach. She fit what some researchers have described as "normal-weight obese syndrome" and "preobesity." Kim had a normal body weight and body mass index (BMI), but a high ratio of body fat to muscle. Her fasting blood sugar appeared normal at 86 mg/dl, but her fasting insulin was elevated at 18 mcIU/ml. Kim's body was secreting large amounts of insulin to keep her blood-sugar level normal.

She enjoyed partying and drinking beer and hard liquor. She ate her lunches at fast-food restaurants and never bothered to exercise. Although her metabolism so far did a good job of burning off her calories, she was an inveterate couch potato and had very little muscle. That's why she was so flabby. She learned that this type of lifestyle would eventually lead to diabetes.

Kim started to improve her eating habits and reduce her intake of alcohol. She also joined a gym and started exercising three days a week. Six months later, while showering, she happened to notice how much firmer her buttocks, legs, and arms had become. Follow-up tests showed that she had substantially increased her muscle mass, and her fasting insulin was now down to 10.2 mcIU/ml. She was happy with the changes and saw her old drinking buddies less and less. She did, however, develop a new network of health-minded friends at the gym.

Practical Guideline #4. Eat High-Fiber, Nonstarchy Fruits

Raspberries, blueberries, blackberries, strawberries, cherries, kiwis, apples, melons, and grapefruit have a lot of vitamins, minerals, and fiber and relatively small amounts of sugars and starches. Include these nutrient-dense foods in your eating plan.

Bananas, dates, figs, grapes, nectarines, oranges, peaches, pears, and plums have far more sugar, and you should not eat these fruits, at least until your weight and blood sugar normalize. Even then, you should limit the quantities of these fruits. In addition, avoid all fruit juices except grapefruit juice and avoid fruit smoothies because they are very high in sugars, but they lack the fiber to buffer their absorption.

Practical tip: Fresh berries are often expensive, so if you can't afford them, opt for frozen. Check the package labels to ensure no sugars have been added.

Practical Guideline #5. Eat Healthy Oils and Fats

We still meet people who believe that all fat is bad and that low-fat or zero-fat diets are the healthiest. The truth is that some fats protect against diabetes and weight gain.

The types of fats stored in your body reflect those in your diet, and people who are overweight or prediabetic usually have unhealthy fat profiles. To correct these undesirable patterns, you must make a point of eating only healthy fats. (Brief definitions are in order. Both fats and oils are more technically referred to as fatty acids. Fats are solid and oils are liquid at room temperature.)

For cooking, use only extra-virgin olive oil and macadamia nut oil, which are high in anti-inflammatory omega-9 fats and relatively low in omega-6 fats and saturated fats. If you need oil for cooking at high temperatures, "light" olive oil and macadamia nut oil have higher smoke points and should work fine.

Emphasize the omega-3 fats found in salmon, tuna, sardines, and other coldwater fish. These fats reduce the insulin response to meals, which reflects an improved insulin function. Fish oils also maintain normal insulin activity, which is otherwise altered by high-fat diets. Some research suggests that eating more fish oils (omega-3s) might help you to lose weight.

Practical tip: Processed and refined foods tend to be high in the omega-6 fats and partially hydrogenated vegetable oils (trans fats). You'll have to read labels carefully to avoid corn, safflower, soybean, and peanut oils and partially hydrogenated vegetable oils. You can replace butter and most cooking oils with olive oil and macadamia nut oils, which are much healthier. Never cook with omega-3 fish oils or cod liver oil.

Practical Guideline #6. Season Your Foods with Herbs and Spices

Culinary herbs—garlic, basil, oregano, rosemary, parsley, dill, saffron, and others—are among the most nutrient dense of all food ingredients. They are rich in vitamins, minerals, and antioxidants, and many herbs have been shown to improve blood sugar. Because culinary herbs are used in relatively small amounts, these health-promoting nutrients will provide only modest benefits, but they will contribute to the broader nutritional advantages of eating healthy foods.

Practical tip: Processed and packaged foods tend to have large amounts of added salt. As you reduce your intake of packaged foods, you will simultaneously lower your intake of sodium. Aside from the nutritional benefits of culinary herbs, they will tantalize your taste buds and counter any belief that healthy foods are boring. Herbs and spices will excite, rather than bore.

Practical Guideline #7. Drink Water and Teas

Thirst is the body's way of demanding water for hydration and maintaining fluid balance. Instead of "boring" water, people often consume soft drinks and coffee—both of which are usually loaded with sugar and caffeine that affect blood-sugar and insulin levels.

Sugary soft drinks have been described as liquid candy. Indeed, the typical 12-ounce can contains about ten teaspoons of sugars, and a 32-ounce cup contains roughly ¼ pound of sugars. Most juices are just as bad, and so are many of Starbucks' and other companies' sweetened beverages.

Artificially sweetened soft drinks may not have the calories, but they have other drawbacks. Some evidence suggests that they alter the brain's appetite centers and lead to a greater consumption of calories. That's on top of the common assumption that a high-calorie meal is fine as long as it's accompanied by a diet cola.

One bright spot in this picture is that in recent years, many people have gotten into the habit of carrying around a water bottle instead of a soft drink. Granted, people pay a premium for bottled water, and the empty bottles fill landfills (if you don't recycle them). But in terms of your health, nothing could be better than simple water.

The research on coffee and diabetes risk is contradictory. Nearly all of the studies showing that coffee either increases or decreases the risk of developing diabetes have been observational, not controlled, so other variables may have influenced the findings. One or two cups of coffee daily may be all right for many people, but the risk of developing multiple health problems increases with greater coffee consumption.

Likewise, research on alcohol consumption is conflicting. Red wine may have some general health benefits, but beer and spirits do not. Alcohol stresses the liver, which breaks down the alcohol. Large amounts of alcohol, as with sugar and carbs, deplete vitamin B1 levels and can lead to a deficiency. If you have prediabetes or diabetes, your liver is already stressed from dealing with sugar and sugarlike carbs, so avoid all alcoholic beverages.

Practical tip: Sparkling mineral water, particularly European brands such as San Pellegrino, Gerolsteiner, Blu, Perrier, and others, is rich in calcium and magnesium. These brands contain hard water (which is good for you), and they have slightly different tastes, based on the mineral content. You can enhance their flavor with a wedge of lemon, lime, or orange.

Iced tea is another option. Regular iced tea contains caffeine, but it also has L-theanine, a natural compound that counteracts the effects of caffeine. Many noncaffeinated herbal teas make great iced teas. Celestial Seasonings' Red Zinger is one of our favorites. Always check the list of ingredients for added sugars, vague "natural sweeteners," or, in the case of one brand, "natural and artificial sweeteners."

Practical Guideline #8. Don't Eat Foods Made with Refined and Added Sugars

Processed and refined foods commonly have added sugars, and in most cases these sugars rapidly increase your blood sugar. The most common sugars are identified on labels as sucrose, high-fructose corn syrup, corn syrup, corn-syrup solids, molasses, maple syrup, dextrose, turbinado sugar, cane sugar, brown sugar, and natural sweeteners. In addition, Xylitol, mannitol, sorbitol, and maltodextrin are sugars, although they are not well absorbed.

Raw sugar is simply dirty white sugar, and brown sugar is white sugar that has been colored with a little molasses—don't be fooled by their more natural look. Many brands of salt also contain small amounts of sugar. So do the most popular sugar substitutes, such as Sweet 'N' Low, Equal, and Splenda. All three contain dextrose, and Equal and Splenda also contain maltodextrin.

Soft drinks and many brands of juice often contain high-fructose corn syrup. Cherry, pomegranate, cranberry, and other juices in natural food stores are often sweetened with grape or apple juice. Although technically more natural, sugar calories are still sugar calories without any other nutritional value.

Honey has the advantage of being so sweet that it's difficult to consume much of it. Still, if you are prediabetic or overweight, it's best to avoid honey as well.

Practical tip: Natural food stores sell several types of noncaloric sweeteners. Our favorite is stevia, which you can buy in liquid or powder form. Stevia is three hundred times sweeter than an equivalent amount of sugar. It's expensive, but a little goes a long way.

Practical Guideline #9. Don't Eat Foods Made with Refined Carbs

Most refined carbs are cereal grains, with cereal grains usually being either wheat or corn. These grain-based carbs include breads, bagels, muffins, pastas, tortillas, and pizza dough. Sometimes soy, rice, and potato flours are used to make breads and pasta. For the flours to be usable, they must be ground to a fine powder, which increases the sugarlike effects of these carbs.

As a general rule, white flour, white bread, white pasta, and white rice are among the most sugarlike carbs. To the surprise of many people, however, whole grains, particularly wheat and corn, are almost as bad in terms of raising blood sugar! All cereal grains are mostly starch, with negligible amounts of other nutrients.

Practical tip: Refined carbs are essentially empty calories, providing virtually no other nutritional value. With two-thirds of Americans overweight, few people can afford to eat empty calories.

Practical Guideline #10. Don't Use Unhealthy Cooking Oils

The most common cooking oils—corn, safflower, cottonseed, soybean, and peanut oil and any type of partially hydrogenated vegetable oil or interesterified fat—increase your risk of developing prediabetes and becoming obese. All of these oils interfere with normal insulin function, thereby altering blood-sugar regulation. Most of these oils, which are high in the omega-6 family of fats, promote weight gain, modify the immune response, and increase your risk of developing inflammatory diseases and diabetic complications.

These cooking oils are relatively inexpensive and are widely used by home cooks and many restaurants. They are found in many processed foods, including salad dressings, mayonnaise, margarine, and baking mixes.

Eating too many saturated fats, such as in fatty, corn-fed meat, isn't good, either. If you're concerned about the saturated fat in eggs, buy eggs fortified with omega-3 fats.

Practical tip: Processed and refined foods are usually high in the omega-6 fats, partially hydrogenated vegetable oils (trans fats), and interesterified fats. You'll have to read labels carefully to avoid corn, safflower, soybean, cottonseed, and peanut oils and partially hydrogenated vegetable oils. If you eat mostly fresh foods, you'll avoid most of the bad oils. (Revisit Practical Guideline #5.)

FOUNDATION FOR HEALTHY EATING HABITS

Five Essential Daily Habits

1. Eat breakfast
2. Eat at regular times
3. Eat slowly and enjoy your food
4. Eat smaller portions
5. Choose your snacks carefully

Six Food-Philosophy Principles for Positive Eating Habits

1. Be mindful of what you eat
2. Eat a diversity of foods
3. Opt for fresh foods
4. Don't take food for granted
5. Don't assume anything about the food you buy
6. Eat organic food as often as you can afford it

Ten Practical Guidelines for Healthy Eating Habits

1. Eat nutrient-dense foods to make every bite count
2. Eat some high-quality protein at every meal
3. Eat plenty of vegetables
4. Eat high-fiber, nonstarchy fruits
5. Eat healthy oils and fats
6. Season your foods with herbs and spices
7. Drink water and teas
8. Don't eat foods made with refined and added sugars
9. Don't eat foods made with refined carbs
10. Don't use unhealthy cooking oils

6

Figure Out What Food Labels Really Mean

We recommend that you eat mostly fresh foods. The reason is simple: fresh foods are almost always more nutritious than processed, refined, and packaged foods. Fresh foods are also much better than processed, packaged foods for improving blood sugar and weight.

You may, however, find it difficult to completely avoid the convenience of prepackaged processed foods. So how do you navigate between packaged foods that are nutritionally acceptable and those that are not?

Before you go food shopping again, it's essential that you learn how to read and decipher the information found on food labels. If you don't take the time to read labels, it's impossible to avoid foods and ingredients that lead to prediabetes and overweight. The situation is a little like getting a new credit card without paying attention to the fine print stating the interest rate. If you ignore the fine print, you could end up paying a steep price.

With food labels, you must distinguish between the advertising that tries to sell you the product and information stating what it actually offers in terms of good or bad nutrition. If you don't read labels, you will pay with your health. Even we have occasionally been victims of a "gotcha" when we took something for granted and skipped reading the fine print.

Learning to Cook—from Scratch

Niki and her husband, Daniel, were both forty-six years old and obese. Three years ago, Daniel's weight ballooned up to four hundred pounds, and he was diagnosed with diabetes. His health continued to deteriorate, and he had difficulty breathing, an inability to walk more than a few feet, and congestive heart failure.

A nutritionist looked at the couple's eating habits and pointed out that they ate few fresh foods. Instead, home-cooked meals consisted of processed and packaged foods, most of them with large amounts of sugar, sugarlike carbohydrates, and trans fats. Because Niki worked two jobs (Daniel was not able to work), she often brought home fast foods—burgers, fries, fried chicken, and pizzas.

The nutritionist coached Niki on how to prepare fresh foods—chopping vegetables, baking fish and chicken—and urged them to avoid most starches, aside from those in vegetables. "I've never cooked this way," Niki said, "but I'm learning."

At first, it wasn't easy. Both Niki and Daniel craved the carbs—pastas, pizzas, and breads—they used to eat all the time. But after a few weeks, Niki had lost ten pounds and Daniel had lost twenty. They also looked better, even though they were still seriously overweight.

Niki and especially Daniel have a long way to go, and Daniel's struggle with his blood sugar and weight will be nothing less than an uphill battle. But Niki is positive about their new way of eating, and both she and Daniel continue to follow the nutritionist's advice and eat mostly fresh foods.

If you already have a habit of checking food labels, read this chapter to reinforce what you know and learn some new tips. If you rarely read the fine print on food packages, you may be in for a shock. While some food manufacturers honor both the letter and the spirit of

---

QUICK TIP

Emphasize Fresh Foods

As you learn how to read food labels, you'll soon realize that the majority of foods in supermarkets aren't very healthy. They're loaded with sugar, sugarlike carbs, dangerous trans fats, and way too much salt. So, what do you eat? The simplest approach is to buy only fresh, perishable foods, such as fish, chicken, and vegetables.

---

food-labeling laws, others follow the letter but exploit labeling loopholes with an apparent intent to deceive shoppers. You'll learn more about food labels than you ever imagined.

What Do Food Labels Really Tell You?

The U.S. Food and Drug Administration requires that virtually all packaged foods disclose their contents with a Nutrition Facts box and a list of ingredients. The intent is well meaning: to help shoppers make informed food purchases. Government agencies in many other countries have similar requirements.

We know that making sense of food labels may at first seem like trying to figure out the tiny print in a legal contract. Keep in mind that you've learned to master many complicated tasks and have read many instruction manuals. Food labels are, if you'll excuse the phrase, a piece of cake. By the time you finish reading this chapter, you'll know everything that's necessary to pick healthy foods and reject unhealthy ones.

The Three Parts of a Food Label

Each box, bottle, jar, can, or bag of food contains three blocks of information: the package front, a Nutrition Facts box, and an Ingredients list.

The *package front*, which describes the product, identifies what's in the package but, aside from that, consists mostly of advertising or graphics to catch your attention and persuade you to buy the product. It may contain any number of healthy-sounding statements, including "No Cholesterol," "Whole Grain," "Lite," "Low-Carb," and "No Trans Fats."

Some of these statements may be no-brainers because some foods (such as olive oil) never contained cholesterol or trans fats. Other products may fudge the truth, as we'll explain shortly. Statements on the front of the box will usually identify what the product contains, such as peas or salad dressing, but may still be misleading. Take all health claims with the proverbial grain of salt.

The *Nutrition Facts box* (sample pictured on page 119) provides a wealth of useful information about the product. Unfortunately, the information allows for some loopholes. For example, serving sizes may be deceptively small, and trans fats may be present even when the Nutrition Facts box claims that the product is free of them.

The *Ingredients list* identifies, in descending order by weight, most or all of the ingredients that were used to make the product. Some ingredients, such as natural or artificial flavors, are extremely vague and could mean anything from sugar to monosodium glutamate. Similarly, "partially hydrogenated vegetable and/or animal shortening" (from the Ingredients list on Twinkies) is also vague, indicating that it may or may not contain animal fat, depending on how the product happened to be manufactured on a given day.

The Food Label Paradox

The government-mandated Nutrition Facts box and Ingredients list are supposed to help people make smart food choices, but there's a catch. The freshest and healthiest foods—such as vegetables, fruits, fish, and chicken—don't have food labels or ingredient lists. In other words, you're more likely to eat healthier foods if you avoid those that have a Nutrition Facts box and an Ingredients list.

The irony is that a Nutrition Facts box and an Ingredients list amount to red flags, usually indicating that the food has been processed. This doesn't mean the food is always unhealthy, depending on the extent of processing, but that it deserves a close look.

While we were researching food labels and supermarket foods for this book, we were aghast at the huge quantities of foods loaded with sugar, refined starches, trans fats, and way too much salt. Many other nutrition experts agree with our assessment, and we were gratified to learn about a supermarket chain that came to a similar conclusion. Nutritionists at

Hannaford Brothers, a New England supermarket chain, gave twenty-seven thousand food products a rating that ranged from zero to three stars. Three-star foods were the most nutritious, whereas zero stars meant that the foods had no redeeming nutritional value.

More than three-fourths of the Hannaford Brothers supermarket's foods received no stars, including many products that were advertised as being healthy! Problematic foods included Lean Cuisine and Healthy Choice dinners, Campbell's Healthy Request Tomato Soup, V8 vegetable juice, and yogurts with fruit. These and other foods had too much sugar, too much salt, too much trans fat, or not enough vitamins, minerals, or fiber.

Are Labels Confusing?

In 2006, in the *American Journal of Preventive Medicine*, Russell L. Rothman, M.D., reported that two-thirds of people could not correctly multiply or divide food quantities, based on the information on food labels. For example, people had trouble calculating the amount of sugars in 2.5 servings or in a 20-ounce soft drink. Nor could they figure out how many carbohydrates were in a half-bagel, compared with a full bagel.

That's a sad state of affairs, but, to be fair, some food companies don't make it easy for shoppers. We'll give you an example. The Nutrition Facts box on Betty Crocker Original Pancake mix defines a single serving as one-third of a cup of flour. This single serving, according to the Nutrition Facts box, should make three pancakes. That seems pretty straightforward; however, the box doesn't indicate that these would be extremely small pancakes compared with the pancakes people normally eat for breakfast.

Meanwhile, the package's cooking instructions start with a full cup of flour—three times as much as in that single serving—so the listed amounts of calories, carbs, and trans fats should be multiplied by three. The math gets even more convoluted. According to the one-third cup (three-pancake) serving size, a full cup of flour should yield nine pancakes. But the cooking instructions state that a cup of flour will yield only six to seven pancakes. This means that the pancakes are now much bigger than those described in the Nutrition Facts box.

A Food Calculator When You Need One

If you ever want to calculate the amount of sugars, carbs, and trans fats in more than one serving of a packaged food, flip open your cell phone. Nearly all cell phones have built-in calculators. Learn to use yours.

We're not trying to pick on Betty Crocker. Many other companies play a similar game, and so, regrettably, do some health food brands. Tazo sells its Simply Red iced herbal tea with apple and pear juice in 13.8-ounce bottles. The Nutrition Facts box notes that the drink has 19 grams of sugars per 8-ounce serving, but the bottle contains more than one serving but less than two servings. We had to use a calculator to figure out that the whole bottle contained about 33 grams of sugars—almost as much as in a 12-ounce can of Coca-Cola! The apple and pear juices sound natural, but they provide mostly sugars and insignificant amounts of other nutrients.

What the Nutrition Facts Box Tells You— and Doesn't

Let's look at what the information in the Nutrition Facts box means, starting from the top.

Serving Size and Servings Per Container

You'll find the serving size and the number of servings per package located immediately below the words Nutrition Facts. The serving size is typically listed in the form of cups or tablespoons, but it may also be listed as "one bar," "two crackers," or "one slice," depending on the food's form. The weight of the serving is also listed in grams. (There are approximately 454 grams in a pound and approximately 28 grams in an ounce.)

This information may seem straightforward, but the listed serving size is often smaller than what most people would normally eat. For example, we recently noticed that the serving size on a bag of cashews was one-quarter cup. That turned out to be only twenty cashews. Of course, the more you eat, the more carbs, oils, and salt you will consume—a perennial problem with any snack food, including potato chips, pretzels, cookies, and ice cream.

Calories and Calories from Fat

The number of calories refers to one serving size that, again, may be unrealistically small. For example, a two-quart (64-ounce) Coca-Cola Classic defines one serving as 8 ounces, which provides 100 calories and 27 grams of sugars. Eight ounces, however, is less than the amount in a can of Coca-Cola. If you have two 8-ounce glasses, you double the calories to 200 and the sugars to 54 grams. If you drink half the bottle, which is easy to do in an afternoon in the office or while driving in your car, you'll consume 400 calories and 108 grams of sugars—almost a quarter pound of high-fructose corn syrup.

Energy bars are popular, and the Nature Valley Strawberry Yogurt bar provides 140 calories; 30 of those calories come from fat. If you eat two bars, as many people do in quick succession, you'll consume 280 calories, 60 grams of which come from fat. If you double the number of servings, this doubles the amount of calories and fat. If you triple the number of servings, this triples the amount of calories and fat.

Total Fat

The next line in the Nutrition Facts box indicates the total amount of fat, in grams, per serving. The next two to four lines provide a breakdown of that fat. Nearly every product also lists the amount of *saturated fat* and *trans fat* in grams. Some products, such as cooking oils, also list the amount of *polyunsaturated fats* and *monounsaturated fats*. Currently, however, there is no legal requirement to list interesterified oils

Nutrition Facts

Serving Size 1 cup (228g)
Servings Per Container 2

Amount Per Serving	
Calories 250	Calories from Fat 110

	% Daily Value*
Total Fat 12g	18%
Saturated Fat 3g	15%
Trans Fat 1.5g	
Cholesterol 30mg	10%
Sodium 470mg	20%
Total Carbohydrate 31g	10%
Dietary Fiber 0g	0%
Sugars 5g	
Protein 5g	

Vitamin A	4%
Vitamin C	2%
Calcium	20%
Iron	4%

* Percent Daily Values are based on a 2,000 calorie diet. Your Daily Values may be higher or lower depending on your calorie needs:

		Calories:	2,000	2,500
Total Fat	Less than		65g	80g
Sat Fat	Less than		20g	25g
Cholesterol	Less than		300mg	300mg
Sodium	Less than		2,400mg	2,400mg
Total Carbohydrate			300g	375g
Dietary Fiber			25g	30g

(fully hydrogenated vegetable oils). To identify interesterified oils, you'll have to examine the Ingredients list.

Occasionally, as with the yogurt bar example on the previous page, the Nutrition Facts box does not account for all of the fats. For example, that yogurt bar lists 3.5 grams of total fat, of which 2 grams are saturated. What kind of fat accounts for the other 1.5 grams? To figure this out, we looked at the Ingredients list, which includes canola oil. We happened to know that canola oil is mostly polyunsaturated and monounsaturated fats, but the average shopper would not.

Cholesterol

The next line of the Nutrition Facts box indicates the amount of cholesterol, in milligrams (mg) per serving. Yet this information may be a little deceiving. A cholesterol-free product may contain sugars, other refined carbohydrates, or trans fats, each of which can boost your body's production of cholesterol. If you have concerns about your cholesterol levels, pay very close attention to the amount of sugars, carbs, and trans fats in foods.

Sodium

Salt is often added to help preserve foods and to improve what would otherwise be tasteless. It literally tricks your tongue into thinking a food has flavor. Many processed foods contain huge quantities of sodium per serving, which increase substantially if you eat two or more servings. Campbell's Chicken Noodle Soup provides a whopping 890 mg of sodium per serving and 2,225 grams of sodium for a standard 10.75-ounce can. Sodium, of course, may contribute to high blood pressure, and some research suggests that excess salt is a factor in osteoporosis and prediabetes. Therefore, it is best to limit your salt intake, so reject high-sodium foods.

Potassium

Some, but not all, products list the amount of potassium. Potassium is an important nutrient, and it can counter many of the effects of excessive sodium. When the Nutrition Facts indicate that potassium is present, it's a plus. It's even better when the food contains more potassium than sodium.

Total Carbohydrate

Don't let the word *total* mislead you. This line indicates the total amount of carbs (including sugar) per serving, not in the entire package. If you have prediabetes or are overweight, you'll want foods with relatively few total carbohydrates. The next two lines in the Nutrition Facts box indicate the breakdown of those carbs, including the amount of *dietary fiber* and *sugars*. These sugars may be naturally occurring or added. To determine which, look at the Ingredients list. Added sugars will most likely be listed as sucrose, corn syrup, corn syrup solids, fructose, or high-fructose corn syrup.

As an example, consider a can of peaches with 30 grams of total carbohydrates, of which 27 grams are sugars. If the Ingredients list includes high-fructose corn syrup, you know that added sugars account for most of those sugars. You don't need these added sugars. Buy fresh peaches instead and cut them up.

Some foods include a line that lists "sugar alcohols." These sugars are not metabolized like regular sugars, and very small quantities are acceptable. Before buying any product containing sugar alcohols, however, try to find a healthier equivalent product.

Protein

This line indicates the amount of protein in a serving. Protein helps to control your blood sugar, but it cannot counter a large quantity of carbohydrates or sugars. There are also different qualities of protein. Eggs and chicken provide very high-quality protein, whereas soybeans, grains, and nuts provide poorer-quality protein. You'll notice that most packaged foods tend to have large amounts of carbs and sugar and small amounts of protein.

% Daily Value

The Daily Value is the FDA's general recommendation for the amounts of total fat, saturated fat, cholesterol, sodium, total carbohydrate, and dietary fiber that the average person should consume each day. The specific percentages of the Daily Value, per serving, are listed to the right side of the Nutrition Facts box. They're based on eating 2,000 calories each day, which is the number of daily calories suggested for the average man. Most women need only 1,600 calories per day, yet the Daily Value does not calculate the percentages of Daily Value for women. The Daily Value is a very general guideline and does not apply to all people, just as no one shoe fits all people.

EDWARD'S STORY
How He Stopped Snoring and Overcame Sleep Apnea

Edward had been a loud snorer for as long as he could remember, but at age fifty he was diagnosed with sleep apnea. His obstructed breathing disrupted his and his wife's sleep, leaving them tired during the day. Edward was about fifty pounds overweight, with elevated blood sugar and blood fats. He loved to eat pizza, pasta, potato chips, and soft drinks, as well as snack while watching television after dinner.

It turned out that Edward had an allergylike sensitivity to wheat and tomatoes, foods that he ate in one form or another at nearly every meal. Eliminating these foods greatly reduced his snoring and sleep apnea. Both he and his wife began to cut back on high-carb foods and eat more lean protein and vegetables. Dietary changes are often more successful when a spouse also follows them. The couple also stopped snacking in front of the television. As Edward's weight dropped over the next six months, his snoring and sleep apnea diminished. Finally, the problems resolved completely a few days after he began taking melatonin supplements about two hours before bedtime.

Vitamins and Minerals

The Nutrition Facts box also lists the amounts of vitamin A, vitamin C, calcium, and iron per serving. These amounts are not listed in milligrams but as a percentage of the Daily Value.

The Ingredients List: What's Really in the Food You Buy

The Ingredients list, usually located below or next to the Nutrition Facts box, identifies exactly what is in the food, in descending order of weight. What's omitted in the Nutrition Facts box almost always turns up in the list of ingredients.

As one example, a jar of Point Reyes Preserves' Pickled Asparagus (an excellent product!) lists

Asparagus, vinegar, olive oil, lemon juice, onion, oregano, basil, salt, pimento, garlic, black peppercorns.

Pacific Natural Foods' Organic Free-Range Chicken Broth lists

Organic chicken broth (filtered water, organic chicken), organic chicken flavor, natural chicken flavor (chicken broth, salt), organic cane sweetener, autolyzed yeast extract, organic onion powder, turmeric, natural flavor.

The ingredients in parentheses identify what the preceding ingredient consists of, if it happens to contain multiple ingredients, such as in the case of

Organic chicken broth (filtered water, organic chicken).

There's no nutritional reason why some processed foods contain thirty, forty, or even a hundred ingredients. Such large numbers of ingredients reflect the needs of large-scale food manufacturing processes, which make products that can be cooked in huge quantities without clogging the equipment and can be divided, packaged, reheated, and still look good and taste fairly appetizing.

In this respect, one of the worst examples we found was Stouffer's Lean Cuisine Chicken, Spinach, and Mushroom Panini, which contained more than a hundred ingredients, although a few are listed more than once. The main ingredients are bread, grilled white meat chicken, low-fat mozzarella cheese, asiago cheese sauce, spinach, mushrooms, red pepper, romano, parmesano and asiago cheese blend, and flavored oil. Here's how the full ingredient list on the box read:

Ingredients: *bread* (bleached enriched flour [wheat flour, niacin, reduced iron, thiamin mononitrate, riboflavin, folic acid], malted barley flour, water, oat fiber, sugar, dough conditioner [guar gum, calcium carbonate, datem, wheat flour, ascorbic acid, enzymes], salt yeast, sodium stearoyl lactylate, sour dough base [bleached enriched flour (wheat flour, malted barley flour, niacin, iron thiamin mononitrate, riboflavin, folic acid), salt, fumaric acid, acetic acid, lactic acid, citric acid, soya oil]), *grilled white meat chicken* (white meat chicken, water, isolated soy protein, modified food starch, chicken flavor [dried chicken broth, chicken powder, natural flavor], sodium phosphate, salt), *low fat mozzarella cheese* ([cultured milk, salt, enzymes], skim milk, modified food starch), *asiago cheese sauce* (water, asiago cheese seasoning [cheese powder] asiago cheese <cultured milk, salt, enzymes>, romano cheese made from cow's milk <cultured milk, salt, enzymes>, cheddar cheese <cultured milk, salt, enzymes>, parmesan cheese <cultured milk, salt, enzymes> salt, lactic acid], whey, creamer [sunflower oil, corn syrup solids, sodium caseinate, mono-& diglycerides, soy lecithin], modified cornstarch, butter flavor [natural flavor, whey, salt, corn syrup solids, butter, guar gum, buttermilk, skim milk solids, annatto & turmeric color], salt, yeast extract, potassium phosphate, lactic acid, xanthan gum, dried garlic, dried onion), *spinach, mushrooms* (mushrooms, water, salt, citric acid, ascorbic acid), *red pepper, romano, parmesan & asiago cheese blend* (romano cheese made from cow's milk [cultured milk, salt, enzymes], parmesan cheese [cultured milk, salt, enzymes], asiago cheese [cultured milk, salt, enzymes]), *flavored oil* (liquid & hydrogenated soybean oil, salt, flavor [soybean oil butter flavor, tumeric & annatto color], lactic acid).

Three Food Ingredients to Always Avoid

Three common food ingredients should always be avoided. They are *partially hydrogenated vegetable oils* (the source of trans fats), *interesterified vegetable oils* (sometimes called fully hydrogenated vegetable oils), and *high-fructose corn syrup* (a blend of sugars). As we explained in chapter 3, trans fats increase weight gain and promote diabetes, whereas high-fructose corn syrup boosts insulin levels and insulin resistance.

Partially Hydrogenated Vegetable Oils Are Often Found in These Types of Foods

Breakfast biscuits

Brownie mixes

Cakes and cake mixes

Cookies

Dinner rolls

Doughnuts

Fish sticks

French fries

Fried chicken

Frozen dinners

Frozen pizzas

Ice cream

Margarine and other butter
   substitutes

Meals in cans

Pancake mixes

Pork and beans

Whipped toppings

Partially Hydrogenated Vegetable Oils Are Found in These Specific Foods

Banquet Crispy Chicken

Banquet Turkey Meal

Betty Crocker Complete
   Meals

Crisco All-Vegetable
   Shortening

DiGiorno Microwave Rising
   Crust Pizza

Duncan Hines Family Style
   Brownies

Eggo Waffles

Hamburger Helper Crunchy
   Taco Flavor

Hungry Man Classic Fried
   Chicken

I Can't Believe It's Not
   Butter

Imperial Margarine

Kraft Shake 'N Bake

Marie Callender's Breaded
   Chicken Parmigiana

Marie Callender's Beef Tips in
   Mushroom Sauce

McCormick Swedish Meat-
   balls Seasoning and Sauce
   Mix

Mission Whole-Wheat Low-Carb Tortillas

Nestle Hot Cocoa Mix

Nutella

Progresso Meals in a Can Italian Style Wedding (meatballs)

Progresso Meals in a Can Potato Broccoli and Cheese

RyKrisp crackers

Skippy Roasted Honey Nut Creamy Peanut Butter

TGI Friday's Onion Rings

High-Fructose Corn Syrup Is Often Found in These Types of Foods

Brownies

Cakes

Candies and candy bars

Chocolate bars

Cookies

Doughnuts

Energy bars

Ice cream

Jellies and preserves

Juices

Ketchup

Pork and beans

Salad dressings

Soft drinks

High-Fructose Corn Syrup Is Found in These Specific Foods

Aunt Jemima Whole Wheat Pancakes

Coca-Cola, Pepsi-Cola, and most other nondiet soft drinks

Hershey's Syrup

Idahoan Butter and Herb Mashed Potato Mix

Kool-Aid Jammers

Kraft Miracle Whip

Kraft Fat-Free Mayo

Kraft Tartar Sauce

Lawry's Herb and Garlic Marinade

Lawry's Sesame Ginger Marinade

Minute Maid Coolers

Ocean Spray Cranberry Sauce

Welch's Concord Grape Jelly

Both Partially Hydrogenated Vegetable Oils and High-Fructose Corn Syrup Are Found in These Specific Foods

Betty Crocker Original
    Pancake Mix

Kellogg's Cocoa Puffs

Mrs. Cubbison's Cheese and
    Garlic Croutons

Ritz Crackers

Twinkies

Beware of the Trans Fat Shell Game

In 2006, the FDA began to require food companies to list trans fats (which are linked to prediabetes and cardiovascular disease) in Nutrition Facts boxes; however, amounts of trans fats that are less than 0.5 (one-half) gram per serving do not have to be listed. In other words, products containing 0.49 gram of trans fats (or less) can be labeled as having zero trans fats per serving. The catch? People can easily consume one or more grams by eating a large serving or two servings.

As an example, the front of the package for Mission brand whole-wheat "carb balance" tortillas states "0g trans fats" in large type, and qualifies that statement with "per serving" in much smaller type. Is the product free of trans fats? While the Nutrition Facts box lists 0 grams, the Ingredients list suggests otherwise, with vegetable shortening and hydrogenated soybean oil prominently mentioned. We don't know anyone who eats just one tortilla at a meal, and our hunch is that two or three of these tortillas provide a substantial amount of trans fats.

The lesson? Even when the Nutrition Facts box states that the food contains no trans fats, look for partially hydrogenated vegetable oils and shortening in the Ingredients list.

It's Not All in the Labels—How Package Sizes Deceive Us

Food companies know that a package's size, shape, and appearance influence what we buy and, just as important, how much we eat. When people buy and eat more food, food companies make more money, so it's in their financial interest to encourage people to eat more, not less.

Each day, the average person makes more than two hundred decisions about food, according to Brian Wansink, Ph.D., a professor of nutrition and marketing at Cornell University in Ithaca, New York, and the author of *Mindless Eating: Why We Eat More Than We Think*. Wansink is one of the sharpest researchers when it comes to eating habits, and he has analyzed how and why people eat in his research laboratory, at parties, and at movie theaters.

Wansink has pointed out that few Americans have a clear idea of what constitutes a normal portion of food. (Europeans and Asians are better at this, and they're often amazed by the quantities of food that Americans eat.) Because people don't have a sense of normal food portions, they look for visual cues in package sizes and what other folks are eating.

Because package sizes have increased for everything from soft drinks to chips, people tend to eat larger quantities than they used to. For example, Wansink has found that people eat almost one-third more ice cream when they're given larger bowls instead of smaller ones. They also eat 53 percent more popcorn from large buckets compared with smaller ones.

The large food packages from Costco, Sam's Club, and Wal-Mart contribute to the problem. When people eat straight from a large container, they just keep eating—not because they're necessarily hungry, but because they lack any visual cues about reasonable serving sizes. When

---

QUICK TIP

Five Ways to Control Portion Sizes

1. Use a teaspoon instead of a tablespoon for soup.
2. Serve dinner on smaller plates.
3. Use small bowls instead of large bowls.
4. Drink from tall skinny glasses instead of short stout ones.
5. Never eat snack foods straight out of a package. Always serve yourself by pouring the food, such as cashews, into a small bowl.

people eat from a small package and the food is gone, it's a signal to stop eating.

Diet Foods That Aren't

Diet food and drinks may be labeled "diet," "low-carb," low-fat," "low-calorie," or "lite." They may (or may not) contain fewer calories than their nondiet counterparts, but they are rarely nutritious products. For example, the many low-fat foods usually contain substantial amounts of sugar and other refined carbs, which the body converts to various types of fats, from triglycerides to belly fat. A diet food is not a license to eat as much as you want.

Most diet foods are highly processed concoctions that were manufactured to be somewhat similar in taste, texture, or function to high-calorie or high-fat foods. For example, many low-carb muffin and pancake mixes use partially hydrogenated vegetable oils to create a buttery texture.

Some brand names, such as Lean Cuisine and Healthy Choice, give shoppers the impression that they are low-calorie or healthier than other foods. In most cases they are only cleverly marketed processed and refined foods. Their relatively small serving sizes are often unrealistic and only whet the appetite, much like an appetizer.

Some evidence suggests that sugar-free soft drinks alter the brain's taste and appetite centers, increasing our desire for sweet foods. But there's another problem with sugar-free soft drinks: people seem to feel that saving a few calories with a diet soft drink makes it permissible to indulge in high-calorie foods such as pizzas.

Organic and Other Natural Foods

Many people believe that organic, natural, and health foods are all about eating only vegetarian foods, such as tofu and bean sprouts. Nothing could be further from the truth.

Natural foods are usually simpler, less-complicated foods and meals. Health foods are any food that's healthy, in contrast to blatantly unhealthy foods. None of this means that natural foods have to taste bad. To the contrary, any good cook relies more on herbs and spices and less on salt and pepper to make a delicious meal. People's taste buds have been numbed by the tastes and textures of processed foods. Natural foods—which are really high-quality foods—have wonderful flavors.

Organic foods are grown without pesticides and with soil-preserving agricultural methods. Several studies have found that organic fruits and vegetables have higher levels of many vitamins, minerals, and antioxidants compared with commercial nonorganic produce. Organic eggs, chicken, beef, and pork come from animals that have been fed grass, organic grains, and no hormones or antibiotics.

Organic foods do cost more, but they are often fresher and tastier than commercially produced foods. A few years ago, the U.S. Department of Agriculture established standards for the labeling of organic foods. As a result, certain terms have specific meanings:

- "100 percent organic" means all the ingredients are organic.
- "Organic" means that at least 95 percent of the ingredients are organic.
- "Made with organic ingredients" means at least 70 percent of the ingredients are organic.

Unfortunately, the term *organic* may sometimes imply a healthier product when it is not. For example, organic bleached white flour and sugar are no better, nutritionally speaking, than nonorganic bleached white flour and sugar.

Meanwhile, the term *natural* is extremely vague and has been abused by both conventional and health food brands. For example, a package of chicken breasts might state "all natural," but that's a little like calling a car an automobile. Again, refer to the Nutrition Facts box and the Ingredients list when deciding on what to purchase.

What Should You Eat?

Eating healthier foods to prevent or reverse prediabetes and to slim down means cooking more fresh foods from scratch and being very selective about what you order in restaurants. (We'll discuss eating out in chapter 9.)

We have already listed many foods that you're better off avoiding. We now want to reintroduce you to the idea of a *food palette*, which Jack described in his book *Feed Your Genes Right*. To explain, artists use a palette to mix colors of paints. Our food palette has a similar purpose: to provide an assortment of foods that you can combine in the kitchen. In chapter 8, we'll describe some basic cooking methods and offer recipes for using the food palette. You'll discover that our food palette is good for your palate!

Protein Sources

These protein sources provide both amino acids and vitamins. They help to lower and regulate your blood-sugar levels. Whenever possible, buy organic, grass-fed, or free-range animal proteins. Select one serving from this group as part of each meal.

Primary protein sources include the following:

Eggs	Turkey
Fish	Shellfish
Chicken	

Optional protein sources include these foods:

Game meats	Lean beef
Hard cheeses	Lean pork
Lamb	Yogurt (sugar free)

Vegetables for Cooking

Vegetables are high in vitamins, minerals, healthy fats, and fiber. Include at least one vegetable—more would be better—with each meal.

Broccoli	Leeks
Carrots	Mushrooms
Cauliflower	Mustard greens
Fennel (anise) bulbs	Onions
Garlic	Shallots
Green beans	Spinach
Kale	

Vegetables for Salads

These vegetables, served cold, are also high in vitamins, minerals, healthy fats, and fiber. Select one, two, or three vegetables from this group each day.

Arugula

Cucumber

Endive

Lettuces, such as Boston
   lettuce or romaine

Radicchio

Spinach

Tomatoes

Watercress

Fruit

These fruits are high in vitamins, minerals, healthy fats, and fiber. Select one, two, or three fruits from this group, as a side dish each day with breakfast or dessert after dinner.

Apples

Blackberries

Blueberries

Cantaloupe

Grapefruit

Honeydew

Kiwifruit

Raspberries

Strawberries

Watermelon

Starchy Foods

Select one, but in a small amount, after your weight and blood sugar normalize. Otherwise, eat extra vegetables.

Legumes

Rice varieties (brown, red,
   purple, and black—not
   white!)

Sweet potato

Wild rice (a grass, not a true
   rice)

Yams

Cooking Oils and Fats

Select one, but use it sparingly.

Butter

Extra-virgin olive oil

Macadamia nut oil

Herb Seasonings

Select one or two, based on recipes and personal tastes.

Basil	Oregano
Bay leaves	Parsley
Cayenne	Rosemary
Cinnamon	Saffron
Dill	Sage
Garlic	Thyme
Herbes de Provence	

Nonherb Seasonings

Although most people do not consider citrus juices to be seasonings, small amounts can "brighten" the flavors of fish, shellfish, chicken, and turkey.

Lemon juice   Lime juice

These seasonings may be used occasionally and sparingly with (but not in place of) the herbs listed above.

Celtic Salt, Cardia Salt, RealSalt, or sea salt

Freshly ground pepper

Beverages

Select one for each meal.

Water: filtered tap or bottled	Tea: black, green, or white
Sparkling mineral water	Herbal tea: hot or iced

What If You're a Vegetarian?

As a general rule, vegetarians have fewer health problems than meat eaters do, in large part because they avoid junk foods and are generally more health conscious. Some vegetarians, however, are pudgy, overweight, and prediabetic. Instead of eating a lot of vegetables, some vegetarians simply avoid animal products and overindulge in breads, pastas, sweets, and sugary drinks.

When vegetarians become overweight and prediabetic, it's usually a sign that their eating habits are a mismatch to their genetics or that they've adopted unhealthy eating habits. To reduce weight and reverse prediabetes, vegetarians must follow one of two dietary plans. First, they must significantly reduce their consumption of grains and sweets and eat more vegetables. Second, they may also have to increase their consumption of dairy products, eggs, fish, or chicken.

Vegetarians generally don't like to hear this advice, in part because they are often addicted to grain products, as are many nonvegetarians. But when vegetarians are overweight or prediabetic, they must consider the possibility that their eating habits may be making them sicker, not healthier.

7

Learn How to Shop at Supermarkets

Today's large supermarkets sell approximately 30,000 to 40,000 food products out of an estimated 300,000 in the total marketplace. The selection is absolutely mind-boggling and the envy of many other nations. The catch is that the vast majority of these foods contribute in big and small ways to people becoming overweight and prediabetic. Your health depends on safely shopping in a nutritional minefield known as the modern grocery store.

You can certainly buy healthy foods at supermarkets, but to do so you have to navigate knowledgeably through aisles full of less-than-healthy products. This task becomes all the more difficult if you live in a small town, where the selection of fresh foods in supermarkets is more limited. Fresh foods, including vegetables, meats, and seafood, are just too difficult and costly to ship to smaller markets. Instead, food distributors ship mostly prepackaged and heavily processed foods and a narrower variety of fruits and vegetables. In other words, you're more likely to have slim pickings in Washington, Pennsylvania, than in Chicago, Illinois.

To be a smart shopper and to fill your cart with healthy foods, it's essential that you understand the meticulously designed layout of modern supermarkets. As a general rule, you'll fare better in a health food or natural food store, but you cannot let your guard down even

---

QUICK TIP

Start with a Shopping List

Always go to the market with a shopping list, and never go shopping when you're hungry. These two steps will greatly reduce the chance of impulse buying and succumbing to sweets and other less-than-healthy foods. For your shopping list, start with a list of the ingredients you'll need to prepare one to three specific recipes.

---

when shopping in the aura of wholesomeness. Many apparently healthy products are loaded with sugar and highly processed carbs, which will only worsen your blood-sugar and insulin levels.

Get Oriented to Your Supermarket

Most supermarkets have a fairly similar layout because of the way that electrical power cables are efficiently laid out for refrigeration. It's simpler from an engineering standpoint to place most refrigerated foods on the perimeter of a supermarket, where wires and pipes are beyond the view of customers. Doing so reduces the cost of running electrical cables and water lines to the center of the store, and many repairs can be made behind the scenes.

Savvy, time-proven marketing also guides the location of foods. Items with the highest profit margins—typically, bakery products and fresh produce—usually greet customers as they walk into the store. Even with the waste and the unsold items, supermarkets make a huge profit from the bakery and the produce sections. As you walk toward the center of the store—you can think of it as the center of a nutritional black hole—you find yourself surrounded by processed and refined foods in boxes, cans, bottles, jars, and bags.

Simplify your shopping. Our recommendations may seem a little challenging at first. That's because you're learning new ways to shop for foods. Keep this in mind: there's a learning curve whenever you tackle something new, and you'll quickly get used to shopping for healthier foods and avoiding junk foods. You'll actually be amazed by how our suggestions will eventually simplify and speed your shopping, mainly because you'll be able to ignore most of the supermarket.

Shop mostly on the perimeter. For better nutrition, shop mostly on the perimeter, where fresh (perishable) and less-processed foods predominate. You'll find fruits and vegetables, meats, eggs, seafood, dairy products, and deli items along the walls. (In contrast, the center aisles are home to most junk foods.) Still, there are perils on the perimeter, so you must always take the time to read food labels. For example, yogurt has evolved from a healthy product to essentially a sugary dessert, and you have to look hard to find unsweetened yogurt.

Look up and down. Product placement within any particular category, be it cereal or detergent, is often determined by slotting fees, a legal form of supermarket bribes. People tend to buy what's at eye level, and food companies pay supermarkets handsomely (tens of thousands of dollars) to place their products at eye level and in other highly desirable locations. You'll often find less expensive, equivalent, and sometimes better products at knee level.

The Different Sections of Supermarkets

Most supermarkets have seven to ten major sections. These are the most common ones.

Produce department. It's hard to go wrong in the produce section as long as you stick to high-fiber, nonstarchy vegetables and fruit. All plant foods contain some starch (carbohydrate), but in so-called nonstarchy vegetables and fruit most of it is in a matrix of fiber. The fiber resists and slows digestion, resulting in a moderate rise in blood sugar and insulin.

High-fiber nonstarchy vegetables include salad ingredients, such as lettuce, tomatoes, and cucumbers, as well as broccoli, cauliflower, spinach, mushrooms, green beans, and many others. High-fiber nonstarchy fruits include blueberries, raspberries, blackberries, strawberries, and kiwifruit. It's best that you avoid or limit your consumption of high-carb potatoes, bananas, and pears.

Personal Boundaries Protect against Stress and Prediabetes

Stress is often overlooked as a contributing factor to prediabetes and overweight. It disrupts eating habits and boosts levels of insulin and cortisol, two hormones that promote belly fat. In Laurie's case, stress sabotaged her lifestyle, and it improved only when she enforced her personal boundaries to buffer stress.

Laurie was an attractive forty-six-year-old, although maybe ten pounds over her ideal weight. She was divorced, had custody of two teenage boys, and managed a real estate office. When she wasn't at work, where she faced constant deadlines, she spent a lot of time driving her boys to and from school and extracurricular sports activities. Laurie was consumed by stress and anxiety because she never seemed to have enough time to do everything, and lunch and dinner usually consisted of fast foods and pizza deliveries. Her social life was zip. Men regularly asked her out to dinner, but she felt too stressed to accept their invitations.

Blood tests showed clear signs of prediabetes. Laurie's fasting blood sugar, insulin, cholesterol, and triglycerides were all elevated. When she was told that the ideal solution was better eating habits, a little more physical activity, and stress reduction, she shook her head and said that stress was just part of her life.

Laurie was referred to both a counselor to address her stress-packed lifestyle and a nutritionist to provide explicit guidance on improving her eating habits. The counselor quickly realized that Laurie had no personal boundaries when it came to work or her teenage boys. She immediately responded to every request and demand made of her. The counselor suggested that Laurie use her lunch hour to detach from the stress over a meal and then go for a short walk. The counselor also advised Laurie to set firm boundaries relating to work and home: not to work overtime or take work home and to let her teenagers know that she needed one uninterrupted hour each night to read and relax.

Meanwhile, the nutritionist provided explicit guidelines on

foods to eat and avoid. She also asked Laurie to reduce her intake of coffee and caffeine-containing soft drinks. Although Laurie was tired for the first few days after cutting back on caffeine, her energy levels rebounded after that. She also had less tension and was less panicky from the usual stresses in her life. Follow-up tests found that her blood sugar, insulin, and blood fats had decreased.

Beware of most prepared salad dressings, though. They often contain unhealthy oils and sugars. You can make great-tasting dressings at home, at a fraction of the cost. We'll explain how in chapter 8.

Dairy department. Although dairy foods generally do not prompt a sharp increase in blood sugar, they do trigger a strong insulin response. Small amounts of European and other hard cheeses, as well as low-fat sugar-free yogurt, should be fine for most people. Western European farmers generally do not inject cows with bovine growth hormone. We do not recommend eating most soft cheeses, such as cream cheese (unless it is organic), Velveeta, or American cheese. If you use milk, half and half, or cottage cheese, buy the organic varieties.

Meat department. As a general rule, we recommend chicken and turkey, although beef, pork, and lamb are acceptable if they are trimmed of excess fat. Even better is meat from free-range, grass-fed, or organically raised animals. You may have to ask your butcher whether the animals were grass-fed but "finished" with grain for the last month or two to add weight and profit. Corn and other grains alter the animals' fat composition, increasing the amount of saturated fat and decreasing heart-healthy omega-3 fats. Game meat, if you like the richer taste, is from free-ranging animals; however, buffalo are now usually fed grain.

Consider paying the extra money for a fresh free-range turkey for your holiday meals. It will cost two to three times more than the well-known brands of frozen turkeys, but it will have an unrivaled flavor. You can order a fresh free-range turkey at most natural food markets.

Seafood department. People love to eat shrimp, but many are wary of other types of seafood. Freshness is a legitimate concern, and, if you ask, the clerk at your fish counter will identify the freshest catch. Don't be embarrassed to ask questions. You should also ask whether the fish is wild or farmed. Wild is healthier and usually higher in omega-3 fats. If you can't afford wild varieties, farmed fish is acceptable. Be sure to rinse all fish under cold water before cooking it.

Many people wonder about mercury contamination in wild fish. Some species, such as swordfish, have high levels of mercury. If you buy fish that are lower on the food chain, you'll have less exposure to mercury. Mercury is toxic only in the absence of selenium, an essential dietary mineral. If you take selenium supplements or get 200 mcg of it in a multivitamin-multimineral supplement, it should protect you. If you eat seafood judiciously, and you can do so two to four times weekly, the benefits outweigh the risks. Pregnant women and small children, however, should still avoid high-mercury seafood.

Other high-mercury seafood includes Atlantic halibut, king mackerel, Gulf Coast oysters, pike, sea bass, shark, swordfish, tilefish (golden snapper), tuna steaks, and canned albacore. Low-mercury seafood includes anchovies, crawfish, Pacific flounder, herring, king crab, sanddabs, scallops, Pacific sole, tilapia, wild Alaska and Pacific salmon, clams, striped bass, sardines, and sturgeon.

Deli counter. As a general rule, sliced chicken, turkey, and beef from the deli counter have fewer noxious ingredients than prepackaged luncheon meats do. You'll be hard-pressed to find much redeeming nutritional value in bologna, salami, and liverwurst.

High-quality deli brands include Applegate Farms, Boar's Head, and Diestel. Avoid presliced meats and cheeses at the deli counter—the clerks preslice them for convenience, but the foods quickly start to turn stale. Ask questions about deli salads. For example, cole slaw often contains sugars.

Bakery. Avoid this department because of the low-nutrient density of the products and because nearly every store-baked product contains sugars and partially hydrogenated vegetable oils. If you want an occasional piece of bread, opt for a European-style dense black bread, which you can find with other prepackaged breads, or La Tortilla Factory's low-carb whole-wheat tortillas. Many prepackaged breads and rolls also contain partially hydrogenated vegetable oils.

Most supermarkets have a separate section with breads, buns, rolls, and tortillas sold in plastic bags. Whole-grain breads might seem healthier, but some are little more than white bread with molasses to give it a brown color. Some breads, brown and white, contain partially hydrogenated vegetable oils.

Hot food department. Many supermarkets sell a variety of hot foods. Chinese and Mexican foods are popular, but many are cooked with unhealthy oils and contain substantial amounts of carbohydrates. The safest hot food is a rotisserie chicken, which you can eat at home with vegetables. Debone the leftover chicken and use it in a salad the next day.

Center aisles. The inner aisles are home to prepackaged foods in boxes, bottles, jars, cans, and bags—highly processed foods with a long shelf life. With a few exceptions, this area of the store contains foods you'll want to avoid because of their high content of sugars, refined carbs, and unhealthy fats. There are very few nutritious foods in these aisles, and skipping them gets you out of the supermarket faster.

Frozen foods. Large freezers are often located between the produce section and the central aisles. The freezers contain frozen dinners, pizzas, ice cream, some juices, and frozen vegetables. As with the center aisles, you have to read package labels very carefully to avoid ingredients that promote prediabetes and overweight.

Navigating Natural Food Stores

As a general rule, natural food stores, such as Whole Foods, Wild Oats, Vitamin Cottage, and the many independent natural food stores, offer more wholesome foods than you'll find in a typical supermarket; however, some so-called natural foods are little more than knockoffs of supermarket products. They may sound and look more healthy, but they can pack plenty of calories, carbs, and sugars.

The natural food and health food industry has long been wedded to whole grains, such as whole-wheat bread. Whole-grain products are more nutritious than refined or enriched products, but they are still primarily sources of starch. Whatever nutrients and fiber exist in whole-wheat or rice bread, pizza dough, or pasta can be obtained in far greater quantities in vegetables.

Always read labels carefully, regardless of where you shop, and wean yourself from hidden sugars. For example, Wild Oats' Organic Limeade might sound like a great drink to quench your thirst, but an 8-ounce glass has 100 calories and 30 grams of sugars—the same as 8 ounces of Coke or Pepsi!

Nature's Choice Multigrain Blueberry Cereal Bars might seem like a quick, healthy breakfast. One bar provides 150 calories and 29 grams of carbs, but more than half of those carbs are pure sugar. Similarly, Nature's Path Apple Cinnamon Toaster Pastries contain 210 calories each, with 18 grams of sugars and 22 grams of other carbs. They're basically desserts masquerading as breakfast foods.

You have to be just as careful with natural cereals. One cup of Wild Oats Performance Crunch Cereal has 230 calories and 39 grams of carbs, of which 20 grams are sugars. The sugars come from evaporated cane juice and brown rice syrup, which are listed in the fine print on the package.

Despite their warm and fuzzy names, soft drinks in health food stores are no better than their supermarket cousins. A 12-ounce can of Blue Sky Natural soda contains 160 calories and 42 grams of sugars from "glucose-fructose syrup," which sounds suspiciously like high-fructose corn syrup. Similarly, a can of Boyland's Cane Cola has 41 grams of sugars.

Health and natural food stores do shine with a great many other products, though. For example, Arrowhead Mills peanut butter contains only peanuts, compared with supermarket brands, such as Skippy, which use partially hydrogenated vegetable oils. Spectrum Naturals uses pressed canola oil, not cheap soybean oil, to make the highest-quality mayonnaise on the market. Blue Diamond Nut Thins crackers are made mostly with ground almonds, pecans, and hazelnuts, and no wheat; they are some of the best-tasting crackers you'll find anywhere.

The main sections of natural food markets and health food stores offer a great bounty, and you'll generally fare better there, nutritionally. Here are some examples.

- The meat department usually sells grass-fed or free-range meats and fowl.
- The deli department normally has high-quality deli meats and prepared salads.
- The seafood department usually has high-quality fresh fish and shellfish.
- The produce department typically sells mostly organic fruits and vegetables.
- The dairy department will likely have organic milk, cream, and other products.

As always, scrutinize the labels of any packaged food to avoid unwanted ingredients.

Other Types of Food Stores

Depending on where you live, you may have access to Italian, Asian, and other types of ethnic grocery stores, as well as boutique food stores. The selections may be varied, exotic, and full of interesting flavors, but don't ever assume anything about ingredients. Make it a habit to read food labels.

Trader Joe's

Trader Joe's, an American grocery chain (now owned by a privately held German corporation), fosters an offbeat but high-quality image. With more than 250 stores in twenty states, Trader Joe's quickly develops a devoted following wherever it opens a new store. The reason is that it carefully selects the products it sells and almost always charges less than identical or comparable products in supermarkets and natural food stores. Trader Joe's has zeroed in on what many people want: generally wholesome, convenient, and comfort foods, along with first-rate customer service.

Trader Joe's sells organic chicken, produce, eggs, and dairy foods alongside more conventional food products. Its cheeses come from both the United States and Europe. Seafood is labeled as to whether it was wild or farmed, as well as the nation of origin. Not everything, however, is low in carbs, sugar, or fats. Trader Joe's has a knack for marketing sweets, and an occasional product contains partially hydrogenated vegetable oils or high-fructose corn syrup. Again, scrutinize the Nutrition Facts box and the Ingredients list of each packaged food.

The Big-Box Stores

Costco, Sam's Club, and Wal-Mart are the big-box stores, so named because of the size of the stores and the size of the food packages they sell. On the positive side, you can buy large quantities of produce, meats, chicken, and fish for a lot less money than the same products will cost you anywhere else. The stores have also begun to take some tentative steps toward stocking organic foods, but time will tell whether their discount-minded customers are willing to pay the difference.

On the negative side, you often get what you pay for. Food manufacturers must take shortcuts to produce foods cheap enough to sell at warehouse prices, and that often means using low-cost, unhealthy ingredients, such as partially hydrogenated vegetable oils and high-fructose corn syrup. As but one example, if you look at the ingredients of corn chips at supermarkets, natural food stores, and Trader Joe's, you'll usually find soybean, safflower, or canola oil. At the big-box stores, it's most often partially hydrogenated vegetable oil. Read the labels extra carefully in these stores.

8

Rediscover the Joy of Cooking

The way you've cooked or have had food cooked for you has been the main factor in your becoming prediabetic and overweight. It's time for you to make a choice—between eating for health and eating for sickness. To improve your health, it's essential that you learn about healthier cooking methods and food ingredients. In this chapter, we'll help you do just that.

We know we're going against the tide. Cooking at home is often considered a chore, and it's certainly no fun if you feel tired after work or have family members who don't appreciate your efforts. Nor is it very inspiring to cook the same old boring foods. Even among people who do enjoy cooking, a lack of time often leads to simply microwaving prepared foods.

Planning meals, shopping, and cooking do take more time than simply driving through McDonald's. But cooking doesn't have to be a chore, and there are many ways to streamline the process so it doesn't take an inordinate amount of time. To be blunt, you can either make the time to cook healthy foods now or plan to be disabled in a few years.

Cooking can be fun, creative, and a wonderful experience that involves all of your senses. You can bring your spouse into the kitchen, share a glass of wine, and talk about your day while you both prepare

QUICK TIP

Organic Beef in a Bag?

Sommers Organic, a leading supplier of cold-case organic meats in the Chicago area, has come up with a convenient and healthy dinner that's available nationwide: lean and tasty beef top sirloin roast and prime rib, precooked and sealed in vacuum-packed plastic bags. All you have to do is boil water in a three-quart pot, then add the bagged meat to reheat it. The whole process takes about ten to fifteen minutes, during which time you can cut and steam some vegetables as a side dish. Sommers products are also sold under the Trader Joe's label, such as "Trader Joe's Fully Cooked and Seasoned Organic Beef Top Sirloin Roast." (You can find more information at www.sommersfare.com, or call 877-377-9797.)

meat and vegetables. Children and teenagers can also help, even if it's just setting the table. Cooking should be considered family time—and a good time to turn off the television and put away cell phones and MP3 players. Relish both the serenity and the activity that make a kitchen a fun place.

Decide What You're Going to Cook

Cooking requires some advance planning. It's not like a fast-food drive-thru where your meal materializes in sixty seconds.

The first step is deciding what you will prepare. If you're at a loss for ideas, look through the recipes in this book, in cookbooks or food magazines, or on the Internet. If it has been a while since you've done any serious cooking, select a simple fail-safe recipe, such as our Mediterranean-Style Pan-Fried Chicken Breasts. Complicated recipes take more time, and they're better left for weekends.

The second step is to make a shopping list for one or two recipes. Look over the ingredients required for the recipe(s), then buy them at the supermarket or the natural food store. You'll want to have certain ingredients in your kitchen all of the time, and you'll also want the right food prep and cooking tools on hand.

Always Have These Ingredients On Hand

Certain food ingredients are important to so many different recipes that it makes sense to have them in your kitchen all the time. They include the following:

Eggs	Dried basil
Extra-virgin olive oil	Dried oregano
Unsalted butter	Peppercorns and a pepper grinder
Fresh garlic	
Lemons	Natural salt, e.g., RealSalt, Celtic Salt, or sea salt
Limes	

Have the Right Tools to Work With

You can't fix a car without a wrench, and you can't sew without a needle and thread. The same rule applies to your kitchen: you need the right tools to get the job done. You may already have a well-equipped kitchen, but if you don't, here are some of the basics you'll need:

- 10- or 12-inch chef's knife, the most versatile knife you'll use
- 4- or 6-inch paring knife for more precise cutting
- Two large plastic cutting boards—the largest size you can fit into your dishwasher
- Large glass or plastic bowl for mixing ingredients
- 8-inch fry pan (skillet), either stainless steel or nonstick
- 12-inch fry pan, either stainless steel or nonstick
- 12-inch nonstick wok
- 1-quart saucepan (also known as a "pot") with a cover
- 2-quart saucepan with a cover
- Heavy-gauge cooking sheet
- Roasting pan with wire rack
- Broiling pan with wire rack
- Aluminum or plastic vegetable steamer basket (inserted into saucepan)
- Heat-resistant plastic spatulas

- Plastic serving spoon
- Food brush (for brushing olive oil)
- Plastic containers of various sizes and lids to store cooked food
- Bleach to clean and disinfect the cutting board and knives after you cut raw meat

Some Basic Cooking Lessons

Many people have forgotten or never learned some of the most basic cooking techniques.

How to Sauté

Sautéing is an easy method of stovetop cooking. It's fast and produces tasty results. The relatively high temperatures help to brown food and seal in moisture. Sautéing quickly evaporates juices near the surface of the meat. That allows the protein to caramelize and form a tasty, slightly firm crust while keeping the inside tender and moist. You can use either a fry pan (skillet) or a wok on a gas stove or an electric range.

You can cook a boneless chicken breast or two, a steak, or seafood in the fry pan. If you're sautéing more than one piece of meat (say, two boneless, skinless chicken breast halves), leave a little room between the pieces. Overcrowding the pan significantly lowers the cooking temperature. When the temperature isn't hot enough, your food steams in its own juices rather than sautés. That's not bad, but sautéing will produce a better taste and texture.

The wok is more suited for small pieces of meat (about the size that you would get in a Chinese restaurant) or shrimp. Again, don't put too much food into the wok at once. The pan can have either a stainless-steel or a nonstick surface—it depends on your preference.

To sauté, preheat the pan or the wok over medium-high heat. When the pan is hot (you can feel the heat rising with your hand), add a little olive or macadamia nut oil (one teaspoon to one tablespoonful) and, if you wish, a pat of butter to enhance browning and taste. The oil and the butter should be hot before you put the meat into the pan. There are two ways to determine whether the temperature is high enough. If you're using butter, simply tip the pan to spread the butter; the butter should sizzle as it swirls across the pan. The other way is to touch the pan with part of the meat or the seafood; if it sizzles on contact, the pan or the wok is hot enough.

Sautéing allows you to season the food while you're cooking (such as sprinkling basil and oregano on chicken) or to add a sauce (such as pesto) when the meat is almost cooked. You can also marinate the meat before sautéing it.

> **QUICK TIP**
>
> ### Chopping Meat and Vegetables
>
> If you're planning to cut up both meat and vegetables for a meal, chop the vegetables first. That way, germs from the meat won't contaminate the vegetables. Likewise, cut up vegetables before chicken and seafood.

How to Pan-Fry

Pan-frying is very similar to sautéing, but we tend to think of it involving relatively larger pieces of meat or fish, such as a boneless chicken breast or salmon fillet. In addition, pan-frying may use a lower temperature and may be particularly suited for cooking a chicken breast that will subsequently be used to make chicken salad. (See the Pan-Fried Chicken Breasts recipe later in this chapter.)

How to Roast and Bake

Roasting is another great way to cook meats, although it takes longer than sautéing. Roasting is like baking but at a slightly higher temperature. For example, roasting is usually done at 400 degrees F (205 degrees C), whereas baking is typically done around 325 degrees F (163 degrees C). A roasting pan enables you to catch the drippings, which you can use to make a sauce, and a well-designed roasting pan will have either a V-shape or a squared-off wire rack that fits above the pan. You'll place the chicken or the beef roast on the rack before it goes into the oven.

How to Broil

Broiling is like indoor grilling—the food is relatively close (within 2 to 3 inches) to the heat source, and the high temperature quickly cooks the food. A broiling pan with a wire rack is a great way to cook burgers and kebabs—the outside gets brown, the inside retains moisture, and excess fat drains off. You have to pay close attention, however, to avoid over-cooking your food.

Most of the time, you can choose between metal or wooden skewers if you're making kebabs with meat, chicken, shrimp, scallops, or vegetables. When using wooden skewers, soak them in water for thirty to forty minutes before using them. Otherwise, they will burn. For kebabs with ground beef or lamb, use metal skewers, preferably those with a flattened surface. You can also spread aluminum foil over the broiling pan (under the wire rack) to simplify clean up.

How to Steam Vegetables

Boiling vegetables takes the life out of them, along with the taste and a lot of the vitamins. A more appealing approach involves steaming vegetables. Steaming is simple, takes five to ten minutes, and makes the vegetables tender but not mushy. You'll need a collapsible vegetable steamer basket, which should cost no more than $5 at supermarkets or cookware stores.

To use the steamer basket (which opens somewhat like a fan), insert it into a 2-quart saucepan; add about an inch of water, so that it barely touches the bottom of the steamer basket; and then add the vegetables. Broccoli, cauliflower, carrots, and other firm vegetables take about seven to ten minutes to cook, while softer vegetables, such as green beans and snow peas, cook in about five to six minutes.

How to Cook Rice

In small amounts, colored varieties of rice make for a tasty and fairly healthy starch. If you're prediabetic, diabetic, or overweight, you must limit these rice varieties to small quantities.

As a general rule, we almost always avoid white rice, except on the occasions when we eat sushi. White rice is about as bland and boring as a food could be. Brown rice, red rice, and purple rice have deeper and more interesting flavors. Just about every natural food store sells long- and short-grain brown rice or brown jasmine rice. Many natural food stores also carry red and purple rice (or you can order them from www.lotusfoods.com). Wild rice is another option, but it is actually a type of grass seed, not a true rice.

Cooking times will vary a little, depending on the variety of rice and your altitude. (Foods take longer to cook at higher altitudes.) Most colored rice will take longer to cook than white rice does. Follow the cooking times given on the package of rice, but make adjustments for the peculiarities of your kitchen. We like to use a combination of either chicken broth or vegetable broth with water, but you can cook rice in water alone.

As a general rule, rinse the rice in a strainer and transfer it to a 2-quart saucepan. Add the broth and/or the water and cover the saucepan. Turn the heat on very high, which should bring the liquid to a boil in about five minutes, then turn the heat down to a simmer. Brown rice should cook fully in about forty minutes, while the red and purple rice varieties will cook in about thirty minutes. When it's cooked, fluff the rice a little with a fork so that it doesn't clump.

Mostly Quick and Easy Breakfasts

Breakfast really is the most important meal of the day, and many people get off to a bad start nutritionally by skipping breakfast. Eating a balanced breakfast—with some high-quality protein, light vegetables, and a little fresh fruit—in our opinion will stabilize your blood sugar for hours. You'll be less tempted to snack on junk foods or overeat during the rest of the day.

If you don't have enough time to make a quick breakfast, it may be because you're too tired to get up early enough to cook. Once you start to eat healthy breakfasts, you'll have more energy in the mornings and will be able to get up fifteen minutes or so earlier to prepare them.

Simple Scrambled Egg   (Serves 1)

½ teaspoon olive oil or small pat of butter
1 large egg
freshly ground pepper
1 teaspoon or so shredded Romano or Parmesan cheese
apple slices

Heat a small nonstick fry pan over medium-high heat. Add the olive oil and continue heating for about 1 minute. Crack open the egg, beat it in a small bowl, and pour it into the fry pan. It will start to set almost immediately. Stir it a little with a heat-resistant plastic spatula and add the pepper. Sprinkle on the cheese and fold over the egg a couple of times. Remove the pan from the heat. Serve the egg with apples slice on the side.

Poached Eggs　　(Serves 1)

Poached eggs will require a few more minutes to prepare, but you won't need any oil or butter to cook them. We have found that specialized egg-poaching pots are usually more trouble than they're worth (unless you're poaching eggs for several people). We've gotten great results using "egg fry rings," which are sold by Williams-Sonoma and other cookware stores. The rings come with a wooden handle, making them easy to use.

splash of white or apple-cider vinegar, optional
2 large eggs

Pour about $\frac{1}{2}$ to 1 inch of water into a medium-size fry pan. If you wish, add a splash of vinegar, which will help the eggs hold their shape. Place two egg rings or cookie cutters in the pan. Bring the water to a simmer. Crack the eggs and pour them into the rings. Let the whites set firmly, about 5 minutes. Cook the eggs for another 1 to 2 minutes, depending on whether you want the yokes soft or solid. At this point, you can remove the rings. When the eggs are cooked, carefully scoop them up with a slotted spoon and transfer them to a plate. If you're allowing yourself some carbohydrates, place the poached eggs over a small amount of warm brown rice or mashed cooked sweet potatoes. They'll taste a lot like eggs on hash browns, only they're healthier.

Hardboiled Eggs　　(Serves 1–2)

2–4 large eggs

Place the eggs in a 1-quart saucepan and add enough water to cover them. Bring the water to a boil, then remove the pot from the burner, cover, and let the eggs set for about 20 minutes. Serve the eggs in a traditional egg cup, or rinse them in cool water and refrigerate and use them the next day. When you crack the eggs open, you can season them with a little sea salt and black pepper as well as a small amount of pesto sauce. You can also dice the eggs and mix them in salads.

Italian-Style Omelet (Serves 1)

1 teaspoon olive oil
2–3 eggs, beaten
2 tablespoons Italian Style Tomato Sauce (see page 159)
1–2 tablespoons shredded Romano, Parmesan, or
 Double Gloucester cheese

Heat a small nonstick fry pan over medium-high heat. Add the olive oil and allow it a minute or so to heat. Pour the eggs into the pan and allow them to set, about 2 minutes. Turn the heat down to medium so the eggs don't burn. When they start to firm a little, use a spatula to lift one side of the omelet a bit, and tip the pan slightly so that some of the liquid egg runs under the omelet. Do the same at the other end of the omelet. (This technique speeds the cooking.) When the top of the omelet becomes gel-like and doesn't readily run, spoon the tomato sauce on one half of the omelet, then sprinkle the cheese on the sauce. Flip over the other half of the omelet so that it covers the tomato sauce and cheese. Remove the pan from the heat and serve the omelet immediately.

Tip: You can also buy high-quality tomato or pasta sauce at your local natural food store.

Ratatouille Omelet (Serves 1)

1 teaspoon olive oil
2–3 eggs, beaten
2–3 tablespoons Quick-and-Easy Ratatouille (see page 183)
1–2 tablespoons shredded Romano, Parmesan, or
 Double Gloucester cheese

Heat a small nonstick fry pan over medium-high heat. Add the olive oil and allow it a minute to heat. Pour the eggs into the pan and allow them to set, about 2 minutes. Turn the heat down to medium so the eggs don't burn. When they start to firm a little, use a spatula to lift one side of the omelet a bit, and tip the pan slightly so that some of the liquid egg runs under the omelet. Do the same at the other end of the omelet. (This technique speeds the cooking process.) When the top of the omelet becomes gel-like and doesn't readily run, spoon the ratatouille on one half of the omelet, then sprinkle the cheese on the sauce. Flip over the other half of the omelet so that it covers the tomato sauce and cheese. Remove the pan from the heat and serve the omelet immediately.

Scrambled Egg and Vegetable Sauté   (Serves 3)

Make this substantial breakfast on a relaxing Sunday morning, eat some of it then, and refrigerate the extra scrambled eggs and vegetables in two covered ramekins. You can reheat one of the ramekins in the microwave oven on Monday morning and the other on Tuesday morning for a quick breakfast.

1 tablespoon olive oil
½ pound fresh mushrooms, sliced
⅓ cup diced scallions (green and white parts)
⅓ cup diced red bell pepper
flavorful sausage, precooked, skin removed, and diced
¼ cup diced artichoke hearts
¼ cup brown rice
4 large eggs, beaten
⅓ cup shredded Romano cheese

Heat a large nonstick fry pan or a wok over medium-high heat. Add the olive oil and about a minute later add the mushrooms, scallions, and bell pepper. Sauté the vegetables a few minutes until they're soft, then add the sausage, artichoke hearts, and brown rice. With a spatula, move the ingredients to one side of the pan and add the eggs to the other side. Allow the eggs to set, about a minute, then use the spatula to mix all of the ingredients. Stir occasionally until the eggs are fully cooked. Depending on the amount of vegetables in the pan, the eggs will cook in 5 to 10 minutes. Remove the pan from the heat and add the cheese and mix well. Use a large plastic spoon to transfer some of the eggs and vegetables to your plate. Transfer the rest to ramekins, cover, and refrigerate.

Super-Fast Blood-Sugar Stabilizers

Nearly everyone, at one time or another, delays or skips lunch because of deadline pressures or other stresses. Skipping a meal—any meal—increases your risk of succumbing to junk foods. It helps to have some handy but healthy options. You can brown bag some of these foods, assembling them either at work or at home the night before. Or, if you're on the road a lot, you can head for a supermarket deli counter instead of a fast-food restaurant.

Fast Blood-Sugar Stabilizer   (Serves 1)

3–4 slices of deli light cheese
3–4 slices of deli turkey or chicken
mustard
1 apple

On a plate or a paper towel, spread 2 or 3 slices of cheese. Put a slice of turkey or chicken on top of each cheese slice. Squeeze a line of mustard on top of the meat, then fold the cheese and meat between your fingers. The apple makes for a nice accompaniment. *Note*: Avoid using salami, bologna, or any other type of heavily processed meat.

Tip: Danish Lite Jarlsburg cheese works particularly well.

Whole-Wheat, Low-Carb Roll-Up   (Serves 1)

This is a good brown-bag lunch, as long as you are not sensitive to the carbs in the tortilla. We often take a couple of these when we have to fly or drive for several hours.

1 whole-wheat, low-carb tortilla
1–2 teaspoons canola mayonnaise (e.g., Spectrum Naturals)
2 slices of cheese, such as lite Swiss
1–2 slices of deli turkey or chicken (or torn pieces of chicken leftovers)
1–2 marinated asparagus spears, optional (from Point Reyes
    Preserves—see resources for details)
mustard

Spread a sheet of aluminum foil on your counter and put the tortilla on top of it. Spread a little mayonnaise on the tortilla, then lay the cheese and meat on top. Add the marinated asparagus spears and drizzle a little mustard on them. Carefully roll the tortilla and wrap the foil around it. Twist the bottom and top of the foil, so that you don't get drippings on your clothes. When you're ready to eat the roll-up, peel away the foil from one tip. Enjoy the roll-ups with tomatoes or pickles on the side.

Cold Plate Lunch   (Serves 1)

Cold meat and cheese plates are often served in Europe, and the most common American version is called antipasto. They're easy to assemble and fun to eat. Instead of bread, try a half-dozen Almond or Pecan Nut-Thins brand crackers. For more information, visit www.bluediamond.com.

2–3 slices or chunks of cheese, such as Cheddar, Brie, Swiss, etc.
2–3 slices of deli turkey, chicken, beef, or ham
sugar-free marinated vegetables, such as mushrooms, asparagus, brussels spouts, carrots, or dill pickles
slices of cucumber, tomato, or avocado
mustard, canola mayonnaise, or horseradish
Nut-Thins brand crackers

Place all of the ingredients on a plate, and enjoy.

Lunch and Other Light Meals

Curried Chicken Salad   (Serves 4+)

Chicken salad doesn't have to be bland and boring. Our recipe will forever change your thinking about this dish.

2½–3 cups (1–1.5 pounds) chicken, cooked, cooled, and diced
1 cup diced celery
½ cup organic raisins
½ cup raw almond slices
1 teaspoon curry powder
¼ teaspoon ground cayenne pepper
1 teaspoon apple-cider vinegar

1 cup canola mayonnaise (e.g., Spectrum Naturals)
salt and freshly ground black pepper

Combine the chicken, celery, raisins, and almond slices in a large bowl and mix them with a fork or a spoon. Sprinkle on the curry powder and ground cayenne pepper and thoroughly mix them in. Now add the vinegar and mix everything to coat the other ingredients. Finally, add the mayonnaise, starting with about ½ cup and adding more to suit your preference for creaminess. Season with salt and pepper. Allow the chicken salad to set in the refrigerator for 1 to 2 hours before serving, to let the flavors integrate. You can substitute diced turkey for the chicken.

Tuna Salad   (Serves 2)

1 can tuna (packed in water, low-sodium preferred)
1 tablespoon roasted, unsalted cashew or almond pieces
2–3 tablespoons canola mayonnaise (e.g., Spectrum Naturals)
2 teaspoons Dijon mustard
salt and freshly ground pepper

Drain the water from the tuna and place it in a bowl. With a fork, break up the tuna into small pieces. Add the nut pieces, mayonnaise, and mustard. Mix the salad well with a fork. Season with salt and pepper.

Lettuce Wrap   (Serves 1)

Lettuce wraps serve as a very low-calorie alternative to whole-wheat, low-carb tortillas. Trader Joe's and some other markets sell packaged lettuce leaves specifically for use as wraps.

2 large leaves of lettuce
some Curried Chicken Salad or Tuna Salad (see previous two recipes)

Fill the furrow of the lettuce leaf with Curried Chicken Salad or Tuna Salad. To eat the wrap, pinch the lettuce leaf so that it doesn't fall apart.

Portobello Personal Pizzas   (Serves 2)

If you miss the taste of pizza, this is a great low-carb alternative. The pieces of ground lamb give it a rich taste.

¼ pound ground lamb
dried basil
dried oregano
1 cup tomato sauce (homemade or good-quality organic sauce)
2 portobello mushrooms, about 5 to 6 inches in diameter
small amount of olive oil
3–6 mozzarella slices (enough to cover each mushroom)

Break apart the lamb into fingertip-size pieces and sauté them in a small skillet over medium-high heat until cooked, 5 to 10 minutes. Sprinkle on the basil and oregano. Remove the skillet from the heat. Drain off the excess fat or soak it up with a crumpled paper towel. Add the tomato sauce and bring it to a boil, then reduce to a simmer, stirring occasionally. You can cover the pan with some aluminum foil to minimize splattering; simmer the tomato sauce to keep it warm.

While the lamb is sautéing, gently rinse the top of the mushroom caps with water and then pat them dry. Remove the stems, break them apart with your fingers, and sauté them with the lamb.

Preheat the oven to 350 degrees F.

Meanwhile, coat the mushroom caps with a little olive oil, spread a tiny bit of olive oil on a cookie sheet, and place the mushrooms gill side up on the cookie sheet. Add the cooked ground lamb to the grill side of the mushroom caps. Bake them for 10 minutes. Remove the cookie sheet from the oven. If the mushrooms have released water, carefully tip them (with a spatula or tongs) to drain off the water, and put them back in the oven for another 1 to 2 minutes. Take the cookie sheet out of the oven, spoon most of the tomato sauce over the mushrooms, lay the mozzarella cheese over the sauce, and spoon the remaining sauce over the cheese. Bake or broil the mushrooms for 1 to 2 minutes. With a large spatula, transfer each mushroom to a plate and serve immediately.

Lamb Burger with Feta Cheese   (Serves 4)

Burgers are usually considered fast food, and lamb is often avoided because it is perceived as particularly fatty. But burgers, prepared correctly, can make an excellent entrée accompanied by healthy side dishes. Ground lamb has a rich taste that makes the best hamburgers pale by comparison. This recipe also drains off excess fat.

1 pound ground lamb
1 clove garlic, diced
3 tablespoons diced parsley
⅓ cup finely crumbled feta cheese
1 teaspoon ground cumin
1 teaspoon ground coriander
extra-virgin olive oil

Place the ground lamb in a large bowl and add the garlic, parsley, feta cheese, cumin, and coriander. Add 1 tablespoon of extra-virgin olive oil. Mix all of the ingredients thoroughly. Form four to six burgers.

Preheat the broiler. Brush olive oil on the wire rack of a broiling pan and arrange the burgers. Place them in the broiler and cook them for about 5 minutes, paying attention that the burgers do not burn. Remove the pan from the broiler and, using a heat-resistant spatula, flip the burgers and put them back in the broiler for another 3 to 4 minutes. Again, make sure they do not burn. When they're cooked, use the spatula to squeeze the excess fat from the burgers. Serve with Tzaziki Sauce and Pan-Fried Eggplant Slices (see the recipes on pages 163 and 187).

Sauces, Pestos, and Marinades

Italian-Style Tomato Sauce   (Serves 4)

This is an easy homemade sauce that you can use with the Portobello Personal Pizza recipe. You can also add some of the sauce to the Mediterranean-Style Pan-Fried Chicken Breasts, especially if you have used basil and oregano to season the chicken.

2 tablespoons olive oil
½ cup diced or chopped mild onions
2–3 garlic cloves, diced
1–3 cups tomato purée or sauce
3–4 tablespoons tomato paste
1 teaspoon dried basil
1 teaspoon dried oregano
1 teaspoon honey

1 bay leaf
sea salt and freshly ground pepper

Heat the olive oil in a 2-quart saucepan over medium heat. Next, add the onion and garlic, stir occasionally, and cook until they're slightly soft. Add the tomato puree/sauce, tomato paste, basil, oregano, honey, and bay leaf. Cover the pan and simmer for 40 minutes. Season with salt and pepper and serve.

Caper Sauce   (Serves 2–3)

This sauce works well with white species of fish, such as sole and halibut. You can also use it with small sautéed pieces of chicken or veal.

½ cup olive oil
⅓ cup capers, rinsed and minced
⅓ cup diced parsley leaves
2–3 tablespoons red wine vinegar
juice of ¼–½ lemon, optional

Heat the olive oil in a skillet over medium heat. Add the capers and parsley, stirring occasionally, and cook them for about 5 minutes. Add the vinegar and allow it to reduce for about 1 minute. If you like lemon, start by adding just a little. Remove the skillet from the heat. Pour the sauce over cooked fish, chicken, or veal.

Piccata Sauce   (Serves 4)

1–2 tablespoons olive oil
1 pat butter
2 garlic cloves, diced
1 medium-size shallot, diced
4 fresh sage leaves, diced; or 1 teaspoon dried sage
½ cup extra dry vermouth or very dry white wine
1 cup high-quality chicken broth, such as Pacific brand
2–3 tablespoons small capers, drained
juice of ½ lemon

Heat a fry pan over medium-high heat and add the olive oil and butter. When the butter melts and sizzles, add the garlic, shallot, and sage, allowing them to sauté for about 2 minutes. Now add the vermouth, letting the alcohol burn off for about 30 seconds or so; then add the chicken broth, capers, and lemon juice. Remove the pan from the heat. You can pour this sauce over chicken strips or seafood, or add the chicken or seafood to the pan and cook them in the piccata sauce.

Mixed Herb Pesto   (Serves at least 4)

Both of these pesto sauces work well with chicken, shellfish, and thick cuts of fish, such as halibut and salmon.

2 cups tightly packed fresh basil leaves, stems removed
½ cup tightly packed fresh parsley leaves, stems removed
½ cup tightly packed fresh mint leaves, stems removed
1 cup tightly packed mixture of chives, cilantro, rosemary, tarragon,
    and thyme leaves, stems removed
½ cup pine nuts
2 garlic cloves, coarsely chopped
⅓ cup grated Romano cheese
1 cup extra-virgin olive oil

All of the herbs should be fresh, clean, and dry to the touch. Place the herbs in a food processor and pulse until they have a pastelike texture. Add the pine nuts and garlic and pulse again. Add the cheese and pulse until the ingredients are thoroughly blended. Now slowly add the olive oil while continuing to pulse and blend it with the ingredients.

Before the oil separates from the rest of the pesto, transfer the pesto with a spatula to the cavities of plastic ice-cube trays. Freeze the pesto overnight; the next day, transfer the cubes to a sealed plastic freezer bag. When you plan to use a couple of the pesto cubes, simply defrost them for a day in the refrigerator or on the countertop for about 1 hour.

Traditional Pesto Sauce   (Serves 4–8)

4 cups tightly packed basil leaves, stems removed
4 ounces pine nuts
4–6 garlic cloves, chopped
1 cup grated Romano cheese
1 cup extra-virgin olive oil

The basil should be fresh, clean, and dry to the touch. Place it in a food processor and pulse until it has a pastelike texture. Add the pine nuts and garlic and pulse again. Add the cheese and pulse until the ingredients are thoroughly blended. Now slowly add the olive oil while continuing to pulse and blend it with the ingredients.

Before the oil separates from the rest of the pesto, transfer the pesto with a spatula to the cavities of plastic ice-cube trays. Freeze the pesto overnight; the next day, transfer the cubes to a sealed plastic freezer bag. When you plan to use a couple of the pesto cubes, simply defrost them for a day in the refrigerator or on the countertop for about 1 hour.

Pesto Aioli   (Serves 2)

An aioli is a mayonnaise flavored with garlic. Use this and other types of aioli as cold dipping sauces for baked salmon, salmon burgers, or crab cakes. We like to start with Spectrum Naturals Canola Mayonnaise, which is sold at most natural food stores. It's healthier and tastes better than other commercial brands of mayonnaise (which use soybean oil).

1 pesto cube, defrosted (see the previous recipes)
2–3 tablespoons canola mayonnaise (e.g., Spectrum Naturals)
1 teaspoon freshly squeezed lemon juice

Place the ingredients in a small bowl and whisk them with a fork. The more lemon you add, the more watery the sauce will be.

Garlic-Rosemary Aioli   (Serves 2)

2–3 tablespoons canola mayonnaise (e.g,, Spectrum Naturals)
1 teaspoon extra-virgin olive oil
1 clove garlic, finely minced
1 teaspoon finely minced fresh rosemary leaves

Place the ingredients in a small bowl and whisk them with a fork.

Olive Tapenade Aioli   (Serves 2)

2–3 tablespoons canola mayonnaise (e.g., Spectrum Naturals)
1 teaspoon extra-virgin olive oil
1 clove garlic, finely minced

1 tablespoon store-bought black olive tapenade
1 teaspoon freshly squeezed lemon juice

Place the ingredients in a small bowl and whisk them with a fork.

Tzaziki Sauce   (Serve with Greek-Style Gyros; yields approximately
3 cups)

1½ cups Greek or other sugar-free yogurt
2 very small cucumbers, diced and seeds removed
2 tablespoons extra-virgin olive oil
2 large garlic cloves, diced
3 tablespoons crumbled feta cheese
½ tablespoon dried dill spice
juice of 1 lemon
salt and freshly ground pepper

In a large bowl, mix all of the ingredients. Season with salt and pepper. For a smoother consistency, use a blender or a food processor.

Rosemary-Garlic Marinade   (Yields approximately ½ cup)

A marinade will season food before you cook it and works especially well with cubed chicken, turkey, beef, or pork. Once the meat is marinated (from 1 hour to overnight), you can sauté the meat or grill it on a skewer. You can also marinate any firm fish, such as tilapia or swordfish, for about 1 hour.

⅓–½ cup extra-virgin olive oil
3 cloves garlic, minced
1 tablespoon minced fresh rosemary leaves
juice of ½–1 fresh lemon
salt and freshly ground pepper
1 pound of meat or seafood

Mix the olive oil, garlic, rosemary, lemon, salt, and pepper in a glass bowl before you add the meat or seafood. If you are sautéing, add some of the marinade ingredients to the pan. If you are grilling, brush the marinade on the skewers before and during (but not after) cooking.

  Tip: If you marinate fish, be cautious when including lemon or lime juice; the juice will start to cook the fish after about 20 minutes.

Salads and Salad Dressings

Vegetable salads (as opposed to pasta and potato salads) provide a wealth of nutrients and fiber. Many people have the best intentions when making or ordering salads, only to be sabotaged by commercial store-bought dressing containing low-quality oils, sugar, salt, and trans fats.

We think most commercial salad dressings are a waste of money, although we do like some of the dressings from Stonewall Kitchens and Annie's. You can make your own tasty salad dressings at home for pennies. Our homemade dressings use vinegar, which, as we explained in chapter 4, can help to improve your blood sugar and reduce your weight.

Greek Cabbage Salad　(Serves 4)

This recipe was adapted from Psisteria Restaurant, Lincolnwood, Illinois.

½ pound finely sliced cabbage (green, red, or blend)
3 tablespoons diced fresh parsley
2–3 tablespoons extra-virgin olive oil
juice of 1 freshly squeezed lemon
½ teaspoon sea salt

In a large glass or plastic bowl, toss the cabbage and parsley with a pair of salad tongs. Drizzle in the olive oil and toss the greens to spread the oil. Add the lemon juice, then the salt, and toss a little more. Allow the ingredients to set in the refrigerator for 1 to 4 hours before serving. Add a little additional lemon juice and sea salt. For convenience, you may use a bag of coleslaw mix. RealSalt and Celtic Salt may be added instead of sea salt.

Cucumber and Lettuce Salad　(Serves 2)

1 romaine lettuce heart
½ English-style cucumber or 2 Persian-style cucumbers
1–2 tablespoons extra-virgin olive oil
1–2 teaspoons lemon juice
sea salt and freshly ground pepper

Thinly slice the romaine heart, beginning at the tip and working toward the base. Transfer it to a colander, rinse under cold water, and then pat it dry with paper towels. Skin and slice the cucumber. Drizzle the olive oil, then the lemon juice over the lettuce, and add a small amount of salt and pepper. Toss all of the ingredients and serve.

Tossed Salad   (Serves 2–3)

Tossed salads are one of the most versatile meals and, aside from a few basic ingredients (e.g., lettuce, tomato, and cucumber), you can add virtually any combination of other vegetables. You'll find that salads actually taste better if you prepare them in a large bowl and toss them with the dressing (instead of adding the dressing at the table). By tossing the salad with the dressing, you can use less dressing because it lightly coats all of the ingredients. That saves a lot of calories, particularly if you use bottled dressing.

BASIC INGREDIENTS
3 cups chopped Romaine lettuce
6–10 cherry tomatoes
1 small cucumber, sliced

OTHER POSSIBLE INGREDIENTS
3 tablespoons diced red bell pepper
2 tablespoons diced scallions
3 tablespoons unsalted cashews or pecans
1 avocado, sliced
4 marinated artichoke hearts, sliced
1 heart of palm, sliced
2 tablespoons pomegranate seeds
$\frac{1}{3}$ cup broccoli or cauliflower florets
$\frac{1}{3}$–$\frac{1}{2}$ cup diced cooked chicken
2 tablespoons shredded Romano cheese

Using salad tongs, mix all of the ingredients before you add the dressing. Toss everything again with the dressing.

Tip: Substitute baby spinach leaves, arugula, or watercress for some or all of the lettuce.

Marinated Mushrooms   (Serves 2–4)

$\frac{1}{2}$ cup extra-virgin olive oil (Kalamata preferred)
$\frac{2}{3}$ cup red wine or balsamic vinegar

2–3 cloves fresh garlic, minced
½ teaspoon honey
⅛–¼ teaspoon sea salt
¼ cup filtered water
⅓ cup finely diced red onion
1 pound fresh small white button mushrooms

In a large bowl, whisk the olive oil, vinegar, garlic, honey, salt, and water. Trim the ends of the mushroom stems, then clean the mushrooms under running water. Add the onions and mushrooms to the marinade and mix them in gently. Refrigerate the mushrooms for several hours before serving.

Mushroom and Cucumber Salad　(Serves 2)

1 head bibb or Boston lettuce
3 Persian-style cucumbers or pickling cucumbers
1 cup of marinated mushrooms (see previous recipe)

Slice or tear apart the lettuce and place the leaves in a large bowl. Peel and slice the cucumbers and add them to the bowl. Add the marinated mushrooms with a little of the marinade as the dressing. Toss and serve.

Greek Salad　(Serves 2–3)

3 cups thinly sliced hearts of romaine lettuce
1 roasted red pepper (from a jar is fine)
10 cherry tomatoes, halved
½ English-style cucumber, sliced
⅓ cup pitted Kalamata olives, sliced (from a can or a jar is fine)
¼ cup chopped scallions (green and white parts)
½ cup crumbled feta or sheep feta cheese
sea salt and freshly ground pepper
2 tablespoons extra-virgin olive oil
2–3 tablespoons red-wine vinegar

Combine all of the ingredients except the salt, pepper, oil, and vinegar in a large bowl and toss. Season them with salt and pepper and toss again. Add the oil and vinegar, toss, and serve.

Pomegranate Salad   (Serves 2)

FOR THE SALAD
1 head bibb or Boston lettuce, sliced
1 head radicchio lettuce, sliced
2 Persian-style cucumbers
10 cherry or grape tomatoes
2 tablespoons pomegranate seeds

FOR THE DRESSING
⅛ cup sugar-free pomegranate juice
⅛ cup sugar-free apple juice
¼ cup extra-virgin olive oil
¼ cup red-wine vinegar

Mix together all of the salad ingredients in a large bowl. Whisk the dressing ingredients in a separate small bowl. Toss the salad with the dressing and serve.

Pomegranate Seeds   (Serves 2–4)

Pomegranate seeds are rich in antioxidants, fiber, other nutrients—and taste. You can sprinkle the seeds on a fruit salad or a green salad. Many people don't know how to prepare a pomegranate for eating, but buying a whole pomegranate is about one-third the price of buying only the seeds.

1–2 pomegranates

It doesn't matter whether the skin feels ripe—the seeds are the edible part. With a knife, cut off the crown and rinse any dirt off the pomegranate skin. Pat it dry and score the skin in quarters. Place the pomegranate in a large bowl with enough water to cover it completely. Use your fingers to pull apart the quarters, then separate the seeds from the rind and the membrane. The seeds will fall to the bottom of the bowl, and most of the small pieces of membrane will float. Discard the pieces of skin and large chunks of membrane. Use a small strainer to scoop up the smaller floating pieces of membranes. Carefully drain the water from the bowl and pick away any remaining pieces of membrane. Transfer the seeds to a plastic storage container, and again drain off any excess water. Refrigerate them until you need them.

These salad dressings are very easy to prepare and will keep for several days in the refrigerator. Vary your dressings with different herbs to keep your salads from getting boring.

Simple Oil and Vinegar Dressing (Yields approximately ½ cup)

¼ cup extra-virgin olive oil
¼–⅜ cup balsamic vinegar
½–1 teaspoon dried basil
½–1 teaspoon dried oregano
juice from ¼ lemon, optional

Combine the ingredients in a bowl and either shake them or whisk them with a fork. You can use the dressing immediately or tightly cover it and refrigerate it for later use. It will keep in the refrigerator for several days. Always shake the dressing before using it because the ingredients will settle or separate.

Apple-Cider Vinaigrette Dressing (Yields ½–¾ cup)

¼ cup extra-virgin olive oil
¼–½ cup apple-cider vinegar
½–2 teaspoons coarse Dijon mustard

Combine the olive oil and vinegar in a bowl and whisk them with a fork. Add a small amount of the mustard, which will thicken the dressing a little. Add more mustard if you'd like a thicker dressing. You can use the dressing immediately or tightly cover it and refrigerate it for later use. It will keep in the refrigerator for several days. Always shake the dressing before using it because the ingredients will settle or separate.

Cherry Vinaigrette Dressing (Yields approximately ¹⁄₁₀ of a cup, enough for 2 servings)

2 tablespoons cherry balsamic vinegar
6 tablespoons extra-virgin olive oil
2 teaspoons fresh lemon juice
2 teaspoons minced shallot
salt and freshly ground pepper

Combine the ingredients in a bowl and either shake them or whisk them with a fork. You can use the dressing immediately or tightly cover it and refrigerate it for later use. It will keep in the refrigerator for several days. Always shake the dressing before using it because the ingredients will settle or separate.

Citrus-Lime Dressing   (Yields approximately 1 cup)

½ cup extra-virgin olive oil
2 teaspoons vinegar, such as balsamic, red wine, or apple cider
2 tablespoons freshly squeezed lemon juice
½ cup freshly squeezed orange juice
6–8 cilantro leaves, finely diced, optional

Combine the ingredients in a blender and adjust the amounts to suit your personal taste. Blend to the desired consistency. You can use the dressing immediately or tightly cover it and refrigerate it for later use. It will keep in the refrigerator for several days. Always shake the dressing before using it because the ingredients will settle or separate.

Main Courses for Dinner

Grilled Shrimp   (Serves 2)

¼ cup extra-virgin olive oil
2 garlic cloves, diced
½ teaspoon ground cayenne or red pepper flakes
juice of ½ lemon
2 tablespoons diced fresh rosemary leaves
2 pounds uncooked shrimp, peeled and deveined (tail on is okay)

You'll need a broiling pan with a wire rack.

In a large bowl, mix together the olive oil, garlic, cayenne, lemon juice, and rosemary. Add the shrimp and toss. Cover, refrigerate, and allow the ingredients to blend for 15 to 20 minutes.

Preheat the broiler. Rub a little olive oil on the wire rack of the broiling pan to keep the shrimp from sticking. (You can do this with your fingers, by wearing plastic kitchen gloves to spread the olive oil, or use a crumpled paper towel dipped in olive oil.) Arrange the shrimp on the wire rack and place the rack and pan 3 to 4 inches under the broiler. Check the shrimp after about 2 minutes—they will turn pink as they cook. With metal tongs, turn over the shrimp. If you have leftover marinade, you can brush it on the uncooked sides of the shrimp. Place the wire rack and pan under the broiler for another 1 or 2 minutes. You can easily adapt this recipe to an outdoor grill, but in either case be careful not to overcook the shrimp.

Shrimp Chipotle Fajitas   (Serves 2–3)

1 tablespoon of either macadamia nut oil or light olive oil
1 medium red onion, thinly sliced
1 large red bell pepper, cored and cut into thin strips
2 tablespoons of Terrapin Ridge Spicy Chipotle Squeeze Garnishing Sauce
1 pound medium or large shrimp, cleaned and deveined
dash of salt
4 La Tortilla Factory low-carb whole-wheat tortillas, optional
grated Cheddar cheese (organic preferred)
sour cream (organic preferred)

Heat a large fry pan over medium-high heat. Add the oil. When it's hot, after about 1 minute, sauté the onions and bell pepper. Add 1 tablespoon of the chipotle sauce. When the onions and pepper have softened, after about 5 minutes, add the shrimp and sauté. Add a dash of salt. After the shrimp start to turn pink, add 1 to 2 more teaspoons of chipotle sauce and continue to sauté until the shrimp are fully cooked. Remove the pan from the heat. If you are using the tortillas, heat them in a microwave oven for about 20 seconds on a medium setting. Serve the fajitas either on a plate or in the tortillas. Add the sour cream and cheese at the table. As an alternative to shrimp, you can use chicken or a firm white fish, such as mahi-mahi, cut into small cubes.

   Tip: Terrapin Ridge Spicy Chipotle Squeeze Garnishing Sauce is available from some specialty grocers or go to www.terrapinridge.com. If it's unavailable, try adding ½ teaspoon of ground dried chipotle peppers.

Shrimp and Scallops in Chanterelle Mushroom Cream Sauce   (Serves 4)

Chanterelle mushrooms have a deep, smoky flavor and a meatlike texture. If you can't find them either fresh or dried, try fresh shitake mushrooms as an alternative.

1 tablespoon olive oil

2 tablespoons butter

6 cloves garlic, diced

2 large shallots, diced

¼–½ cup chanterelle mushrooms (if they're dried, rehydrate
   them in water before cooking)

1½ teaspoons dried basil

1½ teaspoons dried oregano

½ pound medium-size shrimp, cleaned and deveined

½ pound bay scallops

2 tablespoons pine nuts

¼ pint heavy whipping cream

Heat a large fry pan over medium-high heat and add the olive oil and butter. When the butter is melted and sizzling, add the garlic and shallots and sauté them until soft, about 4 minutes. Next, add the mushrooms, basil, and oregano and continue to sauté for a few minutes. Add the shrimp, scallops, and pine nuts and sauté until the shrimp turn pink, 2 to 4 minutes. Add the whipping cream and stir for 1 or 2 minutes. Remove the pan from the heat and serve.

Sautéed Scallops with Saffron Sauce   (Serves 2)

FOR THE SAUCE

⅛ cup dry vermouth (or white wine)

1 cup good-quality chicken broth (e.g., Pacific brand) or fish stock

½ teaspoon or so saffron threads

⅓ cup heavy cream

sea salt and freshly ground pepper

FOR THE SCALLOPS

½ pound bay scallops

¼ lemon wedge

sea salt and freshly ground pepper

Start by making the sauce. Heat a 1-quart saucepan over medium heat, add the dry vermouth, and reduce it by half or so, to evaporate the alcohol. Add the chicken broth. Crush the saffron threads between your fingers and add them to the saucepan. (Wash your fingers with soap after you do this because saffron can stain.) Allow the liquid to reduce by 25 percent, stirring occasionally, 5 to 10 minutes. Add ⅓ cup heavy cream, reduce the heat a little, and stir from time to time. Season with salt and pepper.

While the sauce is reducing, rinse the scallops in a strainer, transfer them to a holding plate, and pat them dry with paper towels. Heat a 12-inch skillet over very high heat, and when it's hot add the scallops. Squeeze the lemon over the scallops, which will offset their fishy smell. Drain off the excess water, stir the scallops around a bit, and sprinkle a little salt and pepper over them. Drain off the excess water again, if necessary. The scallops should cook within 2 to 3 minutes. Lower the heat, add some of the saffron sauce to the skillet, and continue cooking for 1 minute. Remove the pan from the heat and serve the scallops over brown rice. Pour the rest of the sauce over the individual servings of scallops and rice.

Shrimp and Chicken Sausage   (Serves 2–3)

1 precooked 6-inch chicken sausage
olive oil
1 pound shrimp, cleaned and deveined
juice of 1 lemon
1 tablespoon diced parsley
freshly ground pepper

At the market, looked for a savory precooked chicken or turkey sausage. You may use other types of quality sausages, such as Italian sausage, but cook and cool it before starting this recipe.

Remove and discard the sausage skin, then slice or dice the sausage. Next, heat a skillet or a wok over medium-high heat and add 1 tablespoon or so of olive oil. After 1 minute, add the shrimp and stir-fry. Add the lemon juice. When the shrimp start to turn pink, add the diced sausage. Cook until the shrimp are pink on all sides and the sausage has warmed up, 2 to 4 minutes. When serving the dish, you can sprinkle it with the parsley and pepper.

Mediterranean-Style Pan-Fried
Chicken Breasts   (Serves 2)

1 boneless, skinless chicken breast, cut in half (about 1 pound)
1 tablespoon olive oil
seasoning options: dried basil and oregano; fresh diced
    rosemary leaves and garlic; or diced sage leaves

Trim the excess fat and gristle from the chicken. Rinse and pat dry. If the thickness of the breast varies considerably, cut it in half laterally so that the pieces cook more evenly. Heat a skillet over high heat and add the olive oil. When the olive oil is hot, add the chicken. Spread the herbs on the chicken. Cook the chicken for 3 minutes, then turn the pieces over and cook them for about another 3 minutes. When the chicken is done, it will be firm against the pressure of a spatula or the back of a fork. You can slice it through the center to confirm that it is cooked. Remove the pan from the heat and serve.

Pan-Fried Chicken Breasts   (For use in other recipes)

1 boneless, skinless chicken breast, cut in half (about 1 pound)
1 tablespoon olive oil

Trim the excess fat and gristle from the chicken. Rinse and pat dry. If the thickness of the breast varies considerably, cut it in half laterally so that the pieces cook more evenly. Heat a skillet over high heat and add the olive oil. When the olive oil is hot, add the chicken. Cook the chicken for 3 minutes, then turn the pieces over and cook them for about 3 more minutes. When the chicken is done, it will be firm against the pressure of a spatula or the back of a fork. You can slice it through the center to confirm that it is cooked. Remove the pan from the heat and serve.

Pan-Fried Chicken Strips   (Serves 2)

1 boneless, skinless chicken breast
1 tablespoon olive oil
3 garlic cloves, sliced
1 teaspoon dried basil
1 teaspoon dried oregano

Trim the excess fat and gristle from the chicken. Rinse and pat dry. Cut it into strips about ½ inch by 3 inches. Heat a fry pan over medium-high heat, add the olive oil, and about 1 minute later add the chicken. When the chicken is about half-cooked, about 2 minutes, add the garlic, basil, and oregano. Or, instead of these herbs, add some Caper Sauce or Pesto (see the recipes on pages 160 and 161). Cook the chicken for 2 to 3 minutes more, remove the pan from the heat, and serve.

Roasted Whole Chicken   (Serves 3–4)

You will need a roasting pan with a removable wire rack to properly roast a chicken. The chicken will rest on the rack, and the pan will catch the drippings, which you will use for a sauce.

1 whole chicken, 4–5 pounds
1 tablespoon rubbed sage
4 garlic cloves, diced or sliced
1 cup high-quality chicken broth

Preheat the oven to 425 degrees F. Remove the chicken from its plastic wrapping and discard the giblets, which will be tucked inside the cavity. Rinse the chicken inside and out under cold running water, then pat it dry with paper towels. Place the chicken breast side up on the wire rack. With your fingers, loosen some of the skin located above the breast to create a pocket. Rub some of the sage on the breast and under the skin, and rub any extra sage on as much of the chicken's skin as possible. Insert the garlic under the skin and place the extra slices on the bird and in the cavity.

Roast the chicken for about 1 hour. Use an instant-read thermometer to check that the meat in the thickest part of the breast is 160 to 165 degrees. If it isn't that hot yet, continue cooking the chicken for a few more minutes. A larger chicken will need about 10 minutes of additional cooking time per pound of weight. When it's done, transfer the chicken to a serving plate and allow it to rest for 10 minutes to redistribute its moisture. Note that the chicken will continue to cook for a few minutes while resting.

Meanwhile, place the roasting pan (sans rack) over medium heat. Add the chicken broth, bring it to a boil, then turn down the heat to a simmer. With a wooden spatula, scrape the bottom of the pan to loosen the brown bits. Allow the gravy to reduce by about half, stirring it occasionally, about 5 minutes. Slice and serve the chicken and pour the gravy over it.

   Tip: Instead of garlic and sage, use garlic and rosemary.

Tandoori Chicken on a Skewer   (Serves 4)

In India, tandoori chicken is traditionally prepared in a clay tandoori oven; however, you can approximate the flavor in a conventional broiler at home. The spices are rich and exotic, and the simplest approach is to use one of the many commercial tandoori spice mixes, which are usually found next to thyme on the spice rack. Alternatively, use a packet of Asian Home Gourmet Indian Tandoor Tikka mix, available at Asian grocery stores.

1–1½ pounds boneless, skinless chicken breasts, rinsed and
     patted dry, cut into roughly 1-inch cubes
½–¾ cup sugar-free plain yogurt
2–3 tablespoons tandoori spice blend
1 tablespoon extra-virgin olive oil
½ medium sweet onion, very coarsely chopped, optional
½ stick unsalted butter, optional

Place the chicken in a large bowl and add the yogurt, tandoori spice blend, and olive oil. (If you include the onion, add it as well.) Thoroughly mix the ingredients together with your fingers and allow them to marinate in the refrigerator for at least 1 hour or for as long as 8 hours.

   Preheat the broiler.

   Thread the chicken pieces onto metal or wooden skewers. (If you use wooden skewers, soak them in water for 1 hour beforehand to keep them from burning.) If you marinated the onion pieces, use them to separate the chicken cubes. If you like, you can melt the butter in a small dish on the stovetop and brush the butter over the chicken before broiling it and before turning the skewers over.

   Place the skewers on a broiling pan and broil them for about 5 minutes; you can also broil them on an outdoor grill. Turn the skewers over and continue broiling them for another 3 or 4 minutes. Be careful not to overcook them.

Peppermint Chutney   (Serves 4)

Indian chutneys are a cross between relishes and cold sauces. You can use this peppermint chutney as a dipping sauce for tandoori chicken (see the previous recipe) or to spice up any plain piece of cooked fish or chicken. Peppermint leaves seem to work better than other types of mint, and this particular chutney is also a great digestive aid.

1 cup densely packed fresh peppermint leaves
¼ sweet onion, coarsely chopped
2–3 tablespoons water
2 tablespoons fresh lime juice
½–1 teaspoon honey
¼ teaspoon ground cayenne pepper
⅛ teaspoon sea salt

Place all of the ingredients in a food processor and pulse until they are coarsely pureed. Taste the chutney to determine whether you need a little more lime juice, pepper, or water. Keep the chutney refrigerated and covered until you serve it. The chutney is best eaten the day that it's made.

Chicken, Grilled Onions, and Sumac   (Serves 4)

This is a variation of the Grilled Onions with Sumac recipe (see page 186), but is a full meal instead of a side dish.

olive oil
2–3 large red or sweet onions, thinly sliced
1 tablespoon dried sumac spice
1 pound boneless, skinless chicken breasts, rinsed and patted dry, cut into roughly 1-inch cubes
sea salt and freshly ground pepper

Heat a large fry pan over medium-high heat and add a little olive oil when it's hot. Next, add the onions and stir with a spatula to coat them with the oil. After about 5 minutes, reduce the heat to low. Allow the onions to cook slowly and to soften, which may take 30 minutes (depending on the size of the pan and the thickness of the onions. When the onions are soft, add the sumac and stir it to thoroughly mix in the spice. Transfer the onions to a bowl.

Increase the heat to medium-high, add a little more olive oil to the fry pan, and sauté the chicken, about 5 minutes. When the chicken is mostly cooked, add about ½ teaspoon or so of sumac, along with the salt and pepper. Put the onions back into the fry pan and thoroughly mix all of the ingredients. Remove the pan from the heat and serve.

Healthy Chicken Schnitzel   (Serves 2–4)

Chicken schnitzel (in German restaurants) and chicken-fried steaks (in American restaurants) are usually covered with a thick coat of flour and pan-fried in unhealthy oils. Our version uses a light coat of Lotus Foods' Bhutanese Red Rice flour, which quickly browns and has a mouth-watering flavor. For a meal that looks far more exotic, you can use Lotus Foods' Forbidden Rice Flour, which is purple. Both products are available at many natural food stores and at www.lotusfoods.com. (You can also use brown rice flour or potato flour, but they won't produce the rich flavor.)

1–1½ pounds boneless, skinless chicken breasts
1 egg, beaten, in a bowl
¼ cup Bhutanese Red Rice Flour
1 tablespoon olive oil
1 pat butter

Trim any excess fat and gristle from the chicken. Rinse and pat dry. Slice each breast laterally so that it is no more than ¼ to ⅜ inch thick. Dip each piece of chicken in the egg, then dredge it through the rice flour. Heat a large nonstick fry pan over medium to medium-high heat and add the olive oil and butter. When the butter melts and sizzles, start adding the chicken to the pan, being careful not to overcrowd the pan. If the chicken is sliced thin, cook the first side for 2 minutes and the second side for 1 to 2 minutes. Cook thicker pieces of chicken a little longer. Remove the pan from the heat and serve.

Tip: After slicing the chicken, you can pound it thinner. Place the chicken in plastic wrap, folding over the sides several times. Pound the chicken with a food mallet, and dip each piece in egg, then in rice flour. Thinner chicken will cook faster, so be careful not to overcook it.

Saffron Chicken Stir-Fry   (Serves 2–4)

1 teaspoon saffron threads
2 tablespoons water
1 tablespoon olive oil
1 pat butter
4–6 garlic cloves, thinly sliced
1–1½ pounds skinless and boneless chicken breast,
    rinsed and patted dry, cubed
juice of ½ lemon
2 tablespoons heavy cream, optional

Prepare the saffron threads by rubbing them between your fingers and allowing them to soak in about 2 tablespoons of water in a bowl. (Wash your fingers with soap after you do this because saffron can stain.)

Heat a wok or a large fry pan over medium-high heat, add the olive oil and butter, and sauté the garlic for 1 or 2 minutes. Add the chicken and sauté, about 5 minutes. When the chicken is cooked about halfway, add the saffron and water, then add the lemon juice, and continue to sauté until the chicken is cooked. If you wish, add the heavy cream, stir, remove the pan from the heat, and serve.

Camuch   (Serves 2–4)

Camuch is a little like nachos, only better. This variation allows for unique flavors, and you can experiment with different types of meats and cheeses. This meal has a bit more carbohydrates than most of our recipes, so consider it either a very occasional treat or an appetizer if you're having dinner with several other people.

20 unsalted tortilla chips, either blue or yellow corn
salsa, strained of excess water; or Terrapin Ridge Spicy Chipotle
    Squeeze Garnishing Sauce
20 cooked chicken pieces, sliced to about the size of a quarter
20 pieces of cheese, sliced about 1 square inch by ⅛ inch thick
1 cup guacamole

Preheat the broiler. Spread the tortilla chips on a cookie sheet. Dab a small amount of salsa on each chip. Next, place the chicken pieces on top. Place the cheese on top of the chicken. Broil this for 1 to 2 minutes, watching so that the cheese melts but does not burn. Remove the cookie sheet from the broiler. Add 1 teaspoonful or so of guacamole to each chip before serving.

Tip: Good cheeses for this recipe include Red Leicester, Double Gloucester, or any sharp Cheddar.

Greek-Style Gyros

½ pound ground lamb
½ pound ground sirloin or other lean ground beef
1 small sweet onion, grated or finely diced
2 large cloves garlic, finely diced
2 tablespoons fresh diced mint or parsley
1 teaspoon oregano
½ teaspoon cumin
½ teaspoon ground coriander
fresh lime juice

Mix all of the ingredients except the lime juice in a bowl and form into patties. Heat a skillet over medium-high heat or else preheat the broiler. Thin patties are best for pan-frying in olive oil, whereas thicker patties are better for broiling or grilling. When the patties are cooked, about 5 minutes, remove the pan from the heat, squeeze a little fresh lime juice on them, and serve them with Tzaziki Sauce (see the recipe on page 163), brown or jasmine rice, and vegetables on the side. The gyros also go well with Pan-Fried Eggplant Slices (see the recipe on page 187).

London Broil   (Serves 4)

London broil refers to the cooking of flank steak, a lean cut of beef (especially so if it is from an animal that was grass fed). The key is to cook London broil medium-rare, so that it's reddish on the inside but well done on the outside. When overcooked throughout, London broil becomes too dry and tough. You can cook it in a pan, in a broiler, or on a grill.

1–1½ pounds flank steak, sliced about 1 inch thick
dried oregano
fresh diced garlic or Rinaldo's toasted Garlic Gold Nuggets
sea salt and freshly ground pepper

Season both sides of the steak with oregano, diced garlic, salt and pepper.

Heat a pan over high heat (or preheat your broiler or grill). If you're pan-frying, touch the heated pan with the corner of the steak; if the meat sizzles, the pan is hot enough. Sear the flank steak on one side for about 5 minutes, then turn it over and sear the other side for about 4 minutes. Cut the steak in the center to check how well done it is. When it's cooked medium-rare, transfer it to a cutting board or a plate and allow it to rest for 5 minutes to reabsorb its juices. To serve, slice it thinly against the grain.

Salmon Burgers   (Serves 4)

1 pound boneless, skinless salmon fillet
¼ cup diced scallions (green and white parts)
¼ cup diced red bell peppers
1 cup cooked short-grain brown rice or brown sweet rice (which is
     sticky and will help to hold the patties together)
sea salt and freshly ground pepper
1 teaspoon olive oil, optional
fresh lemon juice, optional

Cut the salmon fillet into cubes about 1 inch in size and place them in a food processor. Next, add the scallions, red bell peppers, and rice. Add salt and pepper now or later at the table. Pulse until the ingredients are blended and have the approximate texture of ground beef. Transfer the ground salmon to another bowl.

Heat a fry pan over medium-high heat. (Olive oil probably won't be needed because of the oil in the fish.) With your hands, shape the salmon into patties. (It may help to wear disposable plastic kitchen gloves.) Fry the patties for about 2 to 4 minutes, depending on their thickness; turn them over and fry them for another 1 to 2 minutes. Remove the pan from the heat. Serve the patties immediately or refrigerate them. For added flavor at the table, sprinkle a little fresh lemon juice on the patties or serve them with Traditional Pesto Sauce or Pesto Aioli (see the recipes on pages 161 and 162).

Pan-Fried Salmon   (Serves 1)

You can pan-fry a skinless fillet, but we find that a fillet with skin (on one side) works a little better.

1 salmon fillet, with skin, about the size of your outstretched hand
olive oil
½ teaspoon dried basil
½ teaspoon dried oregano
freshly ground pepper

Season the flesh (nonskin) side of the fillet with a light coating of olive oil, dried basil, dried oregano, and pepper.

Heat a fry pan over medium heat and cook the salmon flesh-side down for 5 to 6 minutes. Turn it over and cook the skin-side down for another 4 to 5 minutes. Cut into the center of the fillet to check that it is cooked. Remove the pan from the heat and serve.

Poached Salmon   (Serves 1–2)

Poaching salmon preserves the fish's own healthy oils without adding any more. Once it's poached, you can serve the salmon with a cream sauce or Pesto Aioli (see page 162). Refrigerate the leftovers, flaking off chunks for salads. Poaching works best with a long, low pot, but you can also use a smaller piece of fish in a 2-quart saucepan.

1-pound fillet of salmon with skin on one side
½ cup white wine or vermouth
1 onion, sliced
1 carrot, sliced
1 bay leaf
1 stalk celery, diced
salt and freshly ground pepper

Fill the pot about halfway or so with water, and add the wine, onion, carrot, celery, bay leaf, and salt and pepper. Bring the liquid to a boil and allow it to simmer for 20 minutes. Meanwhile, wrap the salmon in a strip of cheesecloth. Leave the ends of the cheesecloth long enough to drape over the sides of your cooking vessel—you'll need them to lift the fish out of the water.

Place the cheesecloth (containing the fish) into the simmering water, so that there is 1 to 2 inches of water above the fish. If necessary, add more water. Be careful to keep the ends of the cheesecloth away from the flame or the heating element. Bring the water to a boil again, then reduce it to a simmer. Allow 8 to 10 minutes of cooking time per pound of fish. Grab the ends of the cheesecloth and lift the fish out of the water. With a fork or a knife, check the center to make sure it's cooked. If it isn't, continue poaching the fillet for about 2 more minutes. When it's done, remove the fish from the water and serve with Cream Sauce (see the next recipe) or Pesto Aioli (see the recipe on page 162).

Cream Sauce for Poached Salmon

1 pat butter
1 garlic clove, diced
1 shallot clove, diced
½ cup heavy cream
1 teaspoon dried dill
1 teaspoon coarse Dijon mustard

Heat a small fry pan over medium-high heat, melt the butter, and sauté the garlic and shallots. Add the cream, dill, and mustard. Reduce the heat to a simmer. Remove the pan from the heat. Serve by pouring the sauce over the salmon.

Vegetables and Other Side Dishes

Eggplant Sandwich   (Makes 2–4 sandwiches)

This is actually a vegetable side dish rather than a traditional sandwich; however, the ingredients are ultimately stacked like a sandwich.

1 medium-size eggplant
extra-virgin olive oil
dried basil
dried oregano
roasted red peppers (from a jar)

several slices mozzarella cheese
1 cup tomato sauce
cooked natural, nitrate-free (uncured) bacon, optional

Preheat the broiler.

Rinse the skin of the eggplant, dry it, and cut off the crown. Cut the eggplant in ¼-inch slices, starting from the top to the bottom, so that you end up with slices that measure 2 to 3 inches across at one end and 3 to 4 inches at the other. (Discard the outer slices with the largest amount of skin.)

Brush the slices with olive oil, sprinkle them with basil and oregano, and arrange them on the wire rack of a broiling pan. Broil them for about 5 minutes and turn the slices over with a spatula or tongs. While the eggplant is broiling, heat the tomato sauce in a saucepan or the microwave. Remove the eggplant from the broiler.

With tongs, place slices of roasted red pepper on half of the eggplant slices. Layer the mozzarella cheese on top of the peppers, and put the other "empty" eggplant slices on top of the cheese to create a sandwich. If you like, add a couple of slices of cooked natural, nitrate-free (uncured) bacon to the sandwich. Spread a dollop of tomato sauce over the top eggplant slice. Place the sandwiches in the broiler for 1 minute or so, just to melt the cheese.

Quick-and-Easy Ratatouille   (Serves 4)

2 small eggplants, diced
3–4 tablespoons olive oil
1 large bell pepper, or the equivalent from several
   colored varieties, diced
1 medium red or sweet onion, diced
2 small zucchinis, about 8–10 inches long, diced
4 garlic cloves, minced
1–2 teaspoons dried thyme
1–2 teaspoons dried basil
1 bay leaf
½ cup Italian-Style Tomato Sauce (see page 159)

Because the eggplant takes time to cook and soften, dice it first. Heat a large fry pan over medium-high heat and add about 3 tablespoons of olive oil. Add the eggplant and sauté it while you dice the other vegetables. Keep the pan covered as much as possible to retain the moisture. Next, add the bell pepper, onion, and zucchini. After a few minutes, add the garlic, thyme, basil, and bay leaf. When the vegetables soften, add the tomato sauce. Stir occasionally to keep the vegetables from burning, and keep the pan covered when you're not stirring. Add a little more olive oil if necessary. Turn the heat down and simmer for about 40 minutes. Remove the pan from the heat. Dispose of the bay leaf so that you do not eat it by accident and serve.

Tip: You can also make your own tomato sauce or purchase it from a natural food store.

Steamed Broccoli and Cauliflower   (Serves 2–3)

1 cup broccoli florets
1 cup cauliflower florets

See the section on "How to Steam Vegetables" on page 150. Place the vegetable basket in a 2-quart saucepan and add about 1 inch of water. Place the vegetables in the basket and bring the water to a vigorous boil for 10 minutes. When the vegetables are cooked, remove the saucepan from the burner so that the vegetables don't overcook. Serve them promptly.

Spinach and Leek Sauté

Leeks are related to onions and garlic, but they have a milder flavor. Only the white part is used in cooking.

1 tablespoon olive oil
1 leek, white part only, thinly sliced
one 6-ounce bag fresh baby spinach, stems removed
1 teaspoon toasted garlic pieces (or Rinaldo's Garlic Gold Nuggets)

Heat a large fry pan over medium-high heat and add about 1 teaspoon of the olive oil. Sauté the leek until it's soft, 1 to 2 minutes. Add the rest of the olive oil, then add the spinach and sauté it with the leek. When the spinach starts to wilt, sprinkle on the toasted garlic pieces, sauté every-thing for a few more seconds to thoroughly mix the ingredients, remove the pan from the heat, and serve.

Alternatively, you can use freshly diced garlic. In this case, sauté the garlic for about 1 minute before adding the leek.

Pan-Fried Baby Squash   (Serves 2)

8 finger-size baby zucchini
4 yellow or green custard marrow (another type of small squash)
2 tablespoons olive oil
1 teaspoon dried oregano
1 teaspoon toasted garlic pieces (or Rinaldo's Garlic Gold Nuggets)
sea salt
6 white or crimini mushrooms, sliced
3 tablespoons pine nuts
shredded Romano cheese

Cut off and discard the crowns from the squash. You may, if you wish, slice the zucchini in half (laterally) and slice the custard marrow as well. Heat a skillet over medium-high heat and add the olive oil. When it's hot, after about 1 minute or so, add all of the squash. Sprinkle on the oregano, toasted garlic, and sea salt and sauté, 1 to 2 minutes. Add the mushrooms and sauté another 1 to 2 minutes. When the mushrooms look cooked, add the pine nuts and toast them lightly, stirring con-stantly, for 1 to 2 minutes. Add the Romano cheese—a little or a lot—to suit your taste. Remove the pan from the heat and serve.

Baked Acorn Squash and Garlic   (Serves 2)

Squash is rich in antioxidants, which are good for you, but it also contains a fair amount of carbohydrates. You can substitute baked squash for brown rice so that you don't overdo it on the starches. Use the squash in conjunc-tion with a nonstarchy vegetable, such as broccoli or green beans, with your dinner.

extra-virgin olive oil
1 acorn squash
1 teaspoon toasted garlic pieces (or Rinaldo's Garlic Gold Nuggets)

Preheat the oven to 350 degrees F and lightly coat a baking dish with olive oil. Cut the squash lengthwise (horizontally) down the middle. Use a spoon (a grapefruit spoon works great for this) to remove the seeds. Lightly coat the yellow flesh with olive oil and diced garlic. Alternatively, you can season the squash with Rinaldo's Garlic Gold Nuggets, a brand of toasted garlic in olive oil. Place the two halves of the squash face-down in the pan and bake them for 30 to 40 minutes. Carefully transfer the squash face-up to a dinner plate or a small bowl.

Grilled Onions with Sumac   (Serves 4)

Sumac is a reddish Middle Eastern spice, not to be confused with poison sumac. It adds a pleasant depth of flavor that is very different from that of more familiar spices. You can buy it at Middle Eastern grocers. Use these grilled onions as one of your side vegetables, or slather them over a burger. The only drawback to sumac is that the spice easily sticks between your teeth.

olive oil
2–3 large red or sweet onions, thinly sliced
1 tablespoon dried sumac spice

Heat a large fry pan over medium-high heat, and add a little olive oil when it's hot. Next, add the onions and stir with a spatula to coat them with a little oil. After about 5 minutes, reduce the heat to low. Allow the onions to cook slowly and to soften, which may take 30 minutes (depending on the size of the pan and the thickness of the onions). When the onions are soft, add the sumac and stir it around. Remove the pan from the heat and serve.

Sautéed Spinach and Garlic   (Serves 2)

If you wish, pinch the stems off the spinach a few minutes before cooking.

1 tablespoon olive oil
2–3 cloves fresh garlic, diced
3 ounces (approximately 2 cups firmly packed)
   fresh-bagged baby spinach

Heat a fry pan over medium-high heat and add the olive oil. When the olive oil is hot, after about 1 minute, add the garlic and sauté until it softens, 1 to 2 minutes. Add the spinach and sauté, allowing the spinach to wilt slightly. Remove the pan from the heat and serve immediately.

Pan-Fried Eggplant Slices   (Serves 4)

This side dish goes well with Greek-Style Gyros (see page 179).

1 cup red wine vinegar
¼ cup extra-virgin olive oil
1 tablespoon dried oregano
juice of ½ lemon
1–2 small eggplants

Make the marinade by mixing the vinegar, olive oil, oregano, and lemon juice. Slice the eggplants about ¼-inch-thick horizontally and place them in a bowl with the marinade. Refrigerate, but move the eggplant slices around every 1 to 2 hours to ensure that they soak up some of the marinade. Marinate them for 2 to 4 hours.

Heat a skillet over medium-high heat and place the eggplant slices in the pan to cook for 1 to 2 minutes. Flip them over to cook the other side for another 1 to 2 minutes. When they're done, remove the pan from the heat. Serve with Tzaziki Sauce (see the recipe on page 163).

Greek-Style Sautéed Vegetables   (Serves 2–3)

2 small eggplants
1 red onion
2 tablespoons olive oil
salt
1 tablespoon dried oregano
1 tablespoon dried basil
½ pound sliced mushrooms
1–2 tablespoons apple-cider vinegar
juice of ½ lemon
Greek yogurt or other unsweetened yogurt

Remove and discard the crowns from the eggplants, then chop them into pieces roughly ¼-by-½-inch in size. Chop the onion similarly.

Heat a fry pan or a skillet over medium-high heat and add the olive oil. When the oil is hot (after about 1 minute), add the eggplant and sauté while stirring it with a spatula. Sprinkle a little salt on the eggplant. (We prefer RealSalt or Celtic Salt.) After about 2 minutes, add the onion, followed by the oregano and basil. Cover and allow the vegetables to self-steam for 5 to 10 minutes. Add the mushrooms, mixing them with the eggplant and onion. Add the apple-cider vinegar, followed by the lemon juice. Cover and reduce the heat to a simmer. When the eggplant, onion, and mushrooms have softened, about another 5 minutes, remove the pan from the heat and serve.

After serving the vegetables, spoon a little yogurt on top. This makes a great appetizer or side dish.

Brown, Red, or Purple Rice   (Serves 4–6)

1 cup rice
1 cup good-quality chicken or vegetable broth
   (such as Pacific brand)
1 cup filtered water

Rinse the rice in a strainer; transfer the rice to a 2-quart saucepan. Add the broth and water and cover the saucepan. Heat it over very high heat, which should bring the water to a boil in about 5 minutes; then turn the heat down to a simmer. The rice should cook fully in about 40 minutes. When it's done, remove the pan from the heat and fluff the rice a little with a fork so that it doesn't clump. It should be al dente, so do not overcook it.

Tip: As a variation, after about 20 minutes of simmering, add some finely diced shallots, garlic, sweet onions, and a tablespoon of extra-virgin olive oil to the rice.

Wild Rice   (Serves 6)

1 cup wild rice
1 cup good-quality chicken or vegetable broth (such as Pacific brand)
1 cup filtered water

Rinse the rice in a strainer; transfer the rice to a 2-quart saucepan. Add the broth and water and cover the saucepan. Heat it over very high heat, which should bring the water to a boil in about 5 minutes; then turn the heat down to a simmer. The rice should cook fully in 40 to 50 minutes. When it's done, remove the pan from the heat and fluff the rice a little with a fork so that it doesn't clump. It should be al dente, so do not over-cook it.

Snacks and Desserts

Trail Mix   (Serves 4)

¼ pound raw shelled pecan halves (unsalted)
¼ pound roasted shelled peanuts (unsalted)
¼ pound raw shelled pistachios (unsalted)
¼ pound roasted shelled macadamia nuts (unsalted)
¼ pound roasted shelled cashews (lightly salted)
¼ pound organic Thomson raisins

You can change the types of nuts and raisins to suit your personal tastes. We recommend that no more than one of the nut varieties be salted; the salt will transfer to the other ingredients when you mix them. All of the nuts should be out of the shell. Place the ingredients in a large bowl and mix them with your fingers. Transfer the trail mix to several resealable plastic bags. Keep a bag in your car and where you work and refrigerate the rest.

Figs and Almonds   (Serves 2)

2 pitted figs (preferably organic)
8 raw shelled almonds

Figs and almonds are a Moroccan appetizer. Figs are extremely sweet, so eat these as special treats, not on a regular basis. Remove the stem, or use it to nibble on the fig. Eat the almonds between bites of the figs. The fiber and the carbohydrates in the almonds will help to buffer the sugar in the figs.

Dates with Peanut Butter   (Serves 2)

2 Medjool dates
peanut butter

Slice the dates in half lengthwise and remove the pit. With a butter knife, smear peanut butter into the hollow left by the pit. You may also try this with almond butter or cream cheese. We recommend buying organic peanut and almond butter, or cream cheese, at health food stores.

Cantaloupe and Coconut   (Serves 2–4)

½–1 fresh cantaloupe
¼ cup shredded unsweetened coconut

Cube the cantaloupe and place the pieces in a large bowl. Sprinkle on the shredded coconut and toss.

Fruit Salad   (Serves 3–4)

¼–½ cantaloupe, cubed
¼–½ honeydew melon, cubed
¼ cup unsalted walnut pieces
¼ cup raspberries (fresh or defrosted)
¼ cup blueberries (fresh or defrosted)
1 kiwifruit, cubed
½ apple, cubed
¼–½ cup sugar-free yogurt
½–1 teaspoon ground cinnamon

Place three or more varieties of fruit in a bowl, along with the walnuts. You may vary the amounts to suit your personal taste. Add the yogurt and ground cinnamon, then mix everything gently and serve.

9

Navigate Restaurants and Menus

When you cook foods from scratch at home, you have complete control over all of your ingredients. When you eat in restaurants, however, you surrender much of that control to other people. In this chapter, we explain how to choose healthy foods while dining out and thus reduce your risk of developing prediabetes and becoming overweight. We offer guidelines for selecting restaurants, ordering off the menu, asking questions, and requesting substitute ingredients.

Many people eat out for its entertainment value—having a variety of foods to choose from tantalizes the taste buds, and the atmosphere can certainly enhance a date or please the children. More often, however, people eat out to save time, energy, or both, compared with cooking at home.

Studies have found that people eat about one-third more food when they dine with another person. The amount of food that is consumed increases with the number of people around the table. If you eat out with six other people, odds are that you'll eat almost twice as much as you would by yourself. Be mindful of your portions.

STEVE'S STORY
A New Sense of Purpose in Life

When Steve looked at his father's life and then at his own, he saw himself following in his father's footsteps. His dad had diabetes and was showing clear signs of age-related cognitive decline.

Steve's life was not set for favorable change, and as a result he felt trapped by circumstances. His marriage had ended in divorce, he was responsible for a teenage daughter, and his business had taken a downturn. There was no way to nurture his desire for an alternative career in entertainment. He felt sad, disheartened, and depressed. Steve kept eating way too many refined carbs, from sweets to pizzas, and his weight was pushing three hundred pounds. Not surprisingly, his triglycerides were extremely high.

All of this would have been plenty to deal with, but Steve also had hemochromatosis, a disease in which the body stores large amounts of iron. Because of liver damage from the excess iron, his liver enzymes were elevated and his liver function was below normal.

Steve began to follow Dr. Ron's nutritional recommendations, and the most important supplement for him turned out to be alpha-lipoic acid, a natural substance that doctors have used for decades in Germany to treat diabetes. Like other glucose-regulating nutrients (such chromium and biotin), alpha-lipoic acid stabilized Steve's blood sugar, eased his depression, and dampened his carbohydrate cravings.

Over the next few months, Steve's blood-sugar levels improved, as did his liver enzymes. He lost twenty pounds, felt more energetic, and gained a renewed sense of purpose. There were things in his life that Steve knew he probably couldn't change, but he discovered that he could change his eating habits and his health for the better.

The Restaurant Landscape
from Fast to Slow

As a general rule, fast-food restaurants, national chain restaurants, and neighborhood "greasy spoons" serve meals that contain large amounts of sugar, sugarlike carbs, and unhealthy trans fats, food ingredients that contribute to prediabetes and overweight. Chain restaurant menus are practically identical across the country, although minor accommodations may be made for regional tastes. Much of the food served in these restaurants is processed in large manufacturing facilities and shipped frozen to the restaurants, so very little of it is actually fresh.

Fast-food restaurants include (but are not limited to) Burger King, Carl's Jr, Domino's, Hardee's, KFC, McDonald's, Pizza Hut, Subway, Taco Bell, and Wendy's. Our best advice for these restaurants is simple: avoid them! According to a recent article in the *American Journal of Clinical Nutrition*, people who regularly ate at fast-food restaurants, as opposed to any other type of restaurant, were more likely to become overweight over a seven- to ten-year period.

Although one chain has claimed that you can "have it your way," most meals are anything but individualized. They are the result of an assembly line geared more to efficient production and speed than to good nutrition. While it's possible to stick with a salad, the smells of burgers and fries can weaken the willpower of many people. Besides, salad dressings typically use less-than-healthy soybean oil and downright dangerous partially hydrogenated vegetable oils.

Other national chain restaurants include (but again are not limited to) Applebee's, Boston Market, Chili's, Denny's, IHOP, Marie Callender's, Mimi's Café, Olive Garden, Ruby Tuesday, TGI Friday, and Tony Roma. At these restaurants, it's possible to order carefully and find some acceptable entrees; however, you cannot take anything for granted. Much of the menu will likely be off limits if you are trying to control your blood sugar or weight. Be prepared to ask questions about ingredients and food preparation—and to insist on what you want.

Consider Jack's experience at one of these restaurants. He was delayed at an airport where the only restaurant option was TGI Friday. He tried to order a plain broiled chicken breast, but the waiter insisted that he try

QUICK TIP

Care for a Great Pizza, Minus the Dough?

The late Lou Malnati was the son of the man who originated the first thick-crust pizza. The Malnati restaurants in Chicago serve what may be the very best pizza in the country, with a sauce made from cooked plum tomatoes and a high-quality sausage layer (instead of pieces). A few years ago, the Malnati restaurants introduced a crustless pizza that's pretty darn good. You can get it at any of their locations in the Chicago area—or have the restaurant ship it frozen by Federal Express. You'll find more information at www.tastesofchicago.com.

the restaurant's special sauce (which Jack knew was loaded with sugar and probably trans fats). The waiter brought a small cup of the sauce and stood by the table, attempting to talk him into trying it. Jack asked the waiter to take it away and just get him a plain chicken breast. The meal then seemed to take forever to arrive. The waiter apologized and explained that the chef had poured the sauce over it and was cooking another chicken breast. Jack's meal finally arrived—an overcooked, dried-out piece of chicken. The lesson? Unhealthy ingredients and meals are the rule in most of these restaurants, and the staff has little interest in accommodating out-of-the-ordinary requests.

On the other end of the spectrum are more creative—and often more expensive—restaurants. These are sometimes referred to as fusion (that is, a fusion of different cuisines) or nouveau (new) American cuisine restaurants. Typically, they use fresh ingredients, such as chicken, fish, and vegetables, and nearly everything is prepared from scratch in the kitchen (instead of coming out of the freezer or jars and cans). You still have to ask questions when ordering—such as whether the fish is dusted in flour—but chefs at nouveau American restaurants usually accommodate the dietary needs of their customers.

Portion Sizes and Calories

When eating out, people usually want to feel that they are getting real value for their money. Value typically translates to sheer quantity, not quality, and quantities are usually hefty portions. As but one example,

Italian restaurants often overfeed their customers, with servings of pasta or pizza practically falling off the edges of the plates.

A survey of three hundred restaurant chefs across the United States found that the appearance of food, its cost, and customer expectations were the main drivers behind large portion sizes. Half of the chefs said that calories didn't matter, and four out of five chefs served oversize portions.

People in the restaurant business refer to these huge amounts of food as "indulgent" portion sizes. Restaurants generally don't reduce portion sizes, unless high cost becomes an issue. How do you deal with large portions? One way is to share a dish with another person, although some restaurants will charge a dollar or two for the second plate. Another option is to plan ahead of time to take home leftovers, giving you two meals for the price of one.

Ask Questions before Ordering

To stay on an eating plan that prevents or reverses prediabetes and overweight, you'll have to avoid the same foods that you now bypass at the supermarket. Obviously, that means no sugar- and carb-laden foods, such as bread, pasta, pancakes, fries, and desserts.

You'll also have to ask questions about less obvious ingredients and request substitutions to avoid hidden sugar, sugarlike carbs, and unhealthy fats. Some people get a little uncomfortable asking questions, but most restaurants want to please their customers.

At some restaurants, waiters take our requests (such as a burger without a bun, steamed veggies instead of fries) without missing a beat, and the order comes to our tables exactly as we had ordered it. That's service! On a couple of occasions, where pan-fried fish was generally dredged in flour, the waiter let us know that the fish might fall apart without the flour. That was an acceptable risk, and fish sans flour has always been good.

Unfortunately, some restaurant waiters and chefs seem oblivious to the fact that they work in a service business. We often eat in restaurants, and when we encounter poor service or resistance to accommodating our individual dietary preferences, it means that we'll never come back.

Specific Questions You Should Be Prepared to Ask

When navigating menus at restaurants, always be polite, but don't ever take "I don't know" for an answer. If the waiter doesn't know the answer and just stands there, ask him to check with the chef. It's also a good idea to send the breadbasket back the moment it arrives.

In some ethnic restaurants, you might encounter a language barrier or might inadvertently violate some minor custom. For example, Jack has a favorite Middle Eastern restaurant, and he typically orders dinner there without pita bread (too many empty calories) and no tomatoes (because of an allergy). Even after years of being a regular customer, the owner occasionally comes out of the kitchen and tells Jack these foods are good for him. With a smile, Jack always replies, "They're good foods, but they're not good for me!" Declining tortillas in a Mexican restaurant or rice in an Asian restaurant may also evoke strange reactions.

Some of the questions you might ask when ordering are

- Would you hold the bun?
- Are any hydrogenated vegetable oils used in preparing this meal? If they are, ask that olive oil or butter be substituted.
- Instead of fries, mashed potatoes, or baked potatoes, could you substitute steamed veggies, such as broccoli?
- Instead of pasta salad, could you substitute a small green salad or fresh fruit?
- Does the cook use soybean or olive oil? Try to limit soybean oil, although it is impossible to avoid in Asian restaurants.
- What's in the sauce or the gravy? Many sauces have sugar, flour, and partially hydrogenated vegetable oils.
- Do the salad dressings contain vegetable oil, such as soybean oil, or olive oil? If they are made with vegetable oil, ask for oil-and-vinegar dressing.
- Would you leave the croutons off the salad?
- Would you bring fajitas but hold the tortillas?
- Is the chicken or the fish breaded, battered, or dusted with flour? Ask that the cook not use flour.

QUICK TIP

Sure Bets When Eating Out

Are you trying to figure out what you can reliably order in a restaurant? You're almost always safe if you order one of these dishes:

- Rotisserie or baked chicken
- Baked, grilled, or pan-fried poached salmon
- Shrimp pan-fried in olive oil and herbs
- Chicken, meat, or seafood grilled on a skewer
- Hamburger, turkey burger, chicken burger, or lamb burger (as long as the restaurant doesn't use bread crumbs, and if you order it without the bun)
- Salads (dark lettuce or spinach) without croutons and with an olive oil–based dressing.

- Do you use MSG, also known as monosodium glutamate? It's most common in Chinese restaurants. Insist that it not be used.
- What does the meal come with on the side? Ask for extra veggies instead of potatoes, rice, or pasta.

Navigating Different Types of Restaurants

Our descriptions cover the most common types of restaurants, along with ordering suggestions to help you get a healthy meal.

As a general guideline, order protein as your entrée. It may be seafood, chicken, turkey, or lean cuts of beef or pork. It can be baked, broiled, poached, sautéed, or skewered. Ask that a vegetable or extra vegetables be substituted for the starch (typically, potatoes or rice). Try to avoid beets, beans, corn, and peas, which tend to have a lot of carbs.

We've ranked the types of restaurants, with four stars (****) indicating those that are generally reliable sources of healthy meals and one star (*) for those that are the least reliable.

Buffet Restaurants*

People enjoy American, Chinese, or other types of buffet restaurants because they typically offer a wide variety of foods at a reasonable price. Unfortunately, buffets give people an opportunity to overeat, especially sugar- and carb-rich foods.

How do buffet restaurants make any money when they serve all that food? Buffets generally have an overabundance of starchy foods, especially at the front of the line. That's not an accident. Starchy foods cost the restaurant much less than meat does, and you're likely to have most of your plate filled by the time you get to the protein at the end of the line.

To eat healthy at an American-style buffet, ignore all of the prepared salads, such as the many varieties of pasta salad and potato salad. They're mostly starch, with a soybean oil–based mayonnaise, and maybe with added sugar and partially hydrogenated vegetable oils. Stick with more conventional salad ingredients, such as lettuce, cucumbers, and tomatoes. Ignore most of the prepared salad dressings and instead ask for a simple oil-and-vinegar dressing. Pass on the array of desserts, again, because of their sugar and trans fats.

Some buffets have a chef carving prime rib, ham, or turkey. If he's stingy and gives you only one slice, and you've already bypassed all the sugary and high-carb offerings, insist on a second slice. After all, you're paying for an all-you-can-eat buffet.

Good rule of thumb: Stick to slices of chicken, turkey, beef, or pork, plus salad greens. Use oil-and-vinegar salad dressing, or eat your salad without dressing. Skip Chinese-style buffets because it's virtually impossible to get just meat and vegetables.

Family-Style Restaurants*

These restaurants, sometimes called greasy spoons, resemble some of the national chain restaurants, such as Applebee's or Denny's. Even when they're locally owned, they tend to rely on a lot of processed, prepackaged, and frozen foods.

As a general rule, breakfast is usually the safest meal, but you'll have to order eggs and avoid hash browns, toast, muffins, pancakes, waffles, and other rich sources of carbohydrates. Ask whether you can get your eggs poached—cooked in water instead of with oil—along with a side of fresh fruit. A second choice is an omelet, again with a side of fresh fruit. Canned fruit almost always has added sugar or high-fructose corn syrup.

For lunch or dinner, scan the menu for baked fish, baked chicken, and salads. Ask the waiter what's fresh—for example, fish or chicken breasts—and ask whether it could be pan-fried in olive oil. Another possibility is a burger or a chicken breast sandwich, minus the bun, with a side of steamed vegetables or fresh fruit. A Cobb salad with oil-and-vinegar dressing on the side, a rotisserie chicken, and baked salmon are also safe bets.

Good rule of thumb: Opt for broiled fish, burgers without buns, and green salads with oil-and-vinegar dressing.

Nouveau American Restaurants****

These restaurants are among our favorites, although their eclectic styles make them difficult to characterize. Sometimes their cuisine is described as new or nouveau American restaurants or fusion cuisine. Some are fish restaurants, others reflect regional tastes, and still others adapt pan-Asian and Southwestern cooking styles in unique ways.

What these restaurants do have in common is fresh ingredients, cooking from scratch, and considerable creativity. They often have a Mediterranean bent, but their chefs mix and match food ingredients and spices from different cuisines. They're usually upscale and may sometimes be on the pricey side, but the quality of the food and the atmosphere are usually worth it. Find out about restaurants like this by reading the local newspaper or magazine reviews or check online reviews.

Good rule of thumb: The cuisine may be very inventive. Ask the waiter about ingredients. Fresh fish is usually a good option.

Steak and Rib Restaurants**

Americans love to eat steak. The problem, nutritionally, isn't usually the steak so much as how it's prepared and what is typically served with it. Many popular steak seasonings contain high-fructose corn syrup or other types of sugar. Ask what's in the seasoning and whether the chef could simply use a rub with salt and pepper or herbs such as oregano and garlic.

Baked, mashed, or fried potatoes (steak fries are just thick french fries) add a huge amount of carbohydrates, and potatoes have a stronger effect on blood sugar than ice cream does. Ask for some other type of vegetable, such as steamed broccoli, cauliflower, or asparagus.

Avoid battered or deep-fried appetizers, such as calamari, shrimp, and onion rings. Soups might be problematic because they may contain flour or noodles.

Some steak houses also serve a chicken or seafood dish. Ask how it's prepared and whether the fish or the chicken is fresh.

Ribs are typically served with a barbecue sauce. This sauce almost always contains added sugar, and it may also use wheat flour and partially hydrogenated vegetable oils. For these reasons, it's best to avoid ordering ribs.

Good rule of thumb: Stick with steaks seasoned only with salt, pepper, and herbs—no spice blends and no sauces.

Seafood Restaurants****

Restaurants that specialize in fresh fish typically offer some of the healthiest meals. Many of these restaurants bake, pan-fry, or poach the fish listed on the menu, and the chefs are usually willing to prepare fish any way you prefer, such as baked with a little olive oil or butter. Ask the waiter to substitute extra vegetables instead of rice, pasta, or potatoes.

It's difficult to go wrong with fish as long as it's fresh and not deep fried. Ask what the freshest fish is and how it's prepared. High-quality fish restaurants take pride in what they serve. Some of the options will likely include salmon, trout, and halibut. Team the fish with a fresh vegetable, such as baked or steamed asparagus.

Good rule of thumb: You should be able to find a lot of choices at quality seafood restaurants. Ask whether the fish is dusted with flour.

Italian Restaurants***

For many people, Italian food means garlic bread, pasta, and pizza—all starchy foods. Indeed, more than four hundred types of pasta can be found in Italian cuisine. Still, Italian foods are among our favorite because healthy options abound.

For entrées, consider various types of baked chicken, chicken or veal marsala, chicken with marinara sauce, chicken piccata, and Caesar salad with chicken. Be sure to ask whether the chicken is breaded or dredged in flour. If it is breaded or dusted with flour, ask that it be prepared plain. Veal marsala and veal piccata are also options, but, again, ask whether the meat can be prepared without a dusting of flour. (In our recipes, we sometimes use a light coating of rice flour, which is not as allergenic as wheat flour.) Fresh fish, shrimp, and scallops are also common entrées in Italian restaurants.

In general, safe sauces include pesto, piccata, and various types of tomato sauces, although sometimes tomato sauces contain added sugar. When wine sauces are used in cooking, most of the alcohol burns off.

When you order salad, ask whether the Italian dressing is homemade. If it isn't, get oil and vinegar or ask that the chef make an oil-and-vinegar dressing with basil and oregano. It won't take him more than a few seconds.

Good rule of thumb: Seafood is a safe bet, as is a chicken Caesar salad (without croutons). Many chicken and meat dishes should be acceptable if they are not dredged in flour.

Greek Restaurants***

Greek food is another favorite cuisine because there are many healthy options. Chicken, pork, or lamb souvlaki is typically cooked on a skewer, sometimes with vegetables. Baked or roasted chicken is usually another healthy choice—sometimes it's listed on the menu as Athenian chicken. Check whether the pan-fried fish or the chicken breast is dusted in flour. Entrées usually come with vegetables and either potato or rice. Ask whether the chef can hold the starch and give you extra vegetables. Light tomato sauces are common with the vegetables in Greek restaurants.

Greek salads are good choices, and homemade Greek dressing usually relies on olive oil, vinegar, and oregano. Gyros meat (typically, a combination of ground lamb and beef) is another tasty option, and some restaurants offer a gyros (pronounced "hero") salad, with some of the meat on a bed of lettuce, along with tomatoes, olives, and feta cheese. You should ask, however, whether bread crumbs were used in preparing the gyros.

Good rule of thumb: You'll do well with most chicken and seafood dinners, as well as with lamb chops.

Middle Eastern Restaurants**

Middle Eastern restaurants are usually small family-owned operations, and the menu reflects the family's personal style of cooking. They typically serve a large number of appetizing dishes with unique spices. But the spellings of similar meals (such as sharwarma versus shwarma) may vary somewhat, and a sharwarma in one restaurant may be very different from that in another restaurant. It's a good idea to ask the waiter to describe the meal and its ingredients.

Sharwarma typically refers to bite-size chunks of chicken, beef, or lamb, grilled on the stovetop in olive oil and spices. It might be served with hummus (made from chickpeas), baba ghanoush (made with hummus and eggplant), and salad—or fries. Ask questions, even when the menu seems to state the obvious.

Another option is a kebab, which refers to chicken, beef, lamb, or shrimp cooked on a skewer. It's hard to do anything bad to food cooked on a skewer; however, some types of kebabs use ground lamb or ground beef. Ask whether bread crumbs were used to hold the ground meat together.

Avoid deep-fried foods, such as falafel. Go easy on the rice and hummus, and skip the pita bread.

Good rule of thumb: Chicken and seafood are usually healthy options, but ask about the ingredients in the sauces.

Japanese Restaurants**

Japanese foods are among the easiest Asian cuisines to navigate. One reason is that traditional Japanese cuisine uses relatively few sauces, although sauces are more common at Japanese grills, where a chef cooks in front of four to six customers.

Avoid tempuras—these are battered and deep-fried shrimp and vegetables. If you order teriyaki salmon or chicken, ask that the sauce come on the side. Teriyaki sauces use sugar, but some restaurants make a light sauce and others make a thick, heavy sauce. Be wary of barbecue sauces as well, because they almost always include sugar.

Although some people are concerned about parasites in raw fish, we think the risk is minimal. Well-trained sushi chefs know how to inspect fish that they prepare for customers. You'll consume fewer carbs by eating sashimi instead of sushi. Sushi refers to raw fish (and occasionally a piece of cooked seafood, such as shrimp or eel) on a thumb-size clump of white rice. Sashimi is just slices of raw fish, such as tuna, yellowtail, or salmon.

Your plate of sushi or sashimi will include a green pastelike horseradish called wasabi. To use it properly, transfer a small amount (about the size of your small fingernail) to a little dish, add some soy sauce, and mix the two ingredients together. If you haven't eaten sashimi or sushi before, start with a small amount of wasabi because it can be pungent in large amounts. Using your fingers, dip the fish into the wasabi-soy sauce mix. Aside from taste, the wasabi has another function—it kills parasites.

Many Japanese restaurants serve miso soup with sushi and with a full meal. The soup, made from a light soybean paste and kelp, is quite good. Japanese dinners typically come with a salad. The dressing is almost always sweet, so ask that it be served on the side. That way you can use it sparingly or dilute it with water, if your choose to use it.

Good rule of thumb: Sashimi is a healthy option. Instead of teriyaki salmon, ask for the fish to be broiled with a little lemon juice.

Chinese, Korean, Thai, and Vietnamese Restaurants*

These Asian cuisines offer interesting and tasty dishes, but many of the sauces contain hefty amounts of sugar, even when you avoid the inevitable sweet-and-sour dishes. Be especially wary if the menu refers to "secret" or "special" sauces. Although some of these sauces might be made at the restaurant, there's a good chance that they're delivered from Asian grocers in large jugs. Some of the sauces contain alcohol in the form of rice wine. (Rice wine for cooking is called mirin.) If you don't want to consume alcohol, be sure to ask the waiter questions about the content of the sauces. Certain dishes are also dusted with flour or are deep fried, so be sure to ask about this as well.

Avoid or minimize noodles and rice. Know that virtually everything will be cooked in soybean oil, which we don't consider anywhere near as healthy as olive oil. Avoid egg rolls, which are deep fried. Some Vietnamese and Thai restaurants offer a type of "spring" or "summer" egg roll that is not deep fried. It's usually stuffed with veggies and cooked chicken, and the wrapper is most often made from rice flour. Served cold, it has a refreshing taste.

Japanese and Chinese rice bowl or express restaurants are the Asian equivalent of fast food. Many people believe that a quick Asian-style lunch is healthier than an American fast-food lunch. The problem is that you get a small amount of chicken, beef, pork, or seafood, often with a sugary sauce, on top of a large mass of white rice.

Of these cuisines, Thai food probably contains the least amount of hidden sugar and other types of carbs. If you're sensitive to dairy foods, Thai cuisine offers a bonus: coconut milk is often used the way other cuisines use dairy. The creamy soups typically use coconut milk with vegetables to create distinctive broths. Noodle dishes tend to use rice noodles—but don't overeat them. Again, ask questions, and go easy on the rice.

Good rule of thumb: Thai food is the best choice, but ask about the ingredients in the sauces.

Mexican Restaurants*

Mexican restaurants are extremely popular—and also problematic. The chips are deep fried, and partially hydrogenated oils may be used to fry the tortillas used in quesadillas or tostadas. If you have food allergies, Mexican foods may serve up a lot of what you're sensitive to, particularly wheat, corn, and dairy.

To navigate the typical Mexican restaurant, order fajitas—grilled chicken or beef, along with onions, bell peppers, and possibly tomatoes. Eat off the plate instead of assembling these ingredients in tortillas. The guacamole is fine, but skip the beans and rice, which have a lot of carbohydrate calories.

Some Mexican and South American–style restaurants serve ceviche, which typically contains seafood marinated and "cold cooked" in lime juice and a mix of mild and hot peppers. Ceviche is very tasty and free of sugar and other carbs. Still other options are *carne asada* (broiled or grilled steak) and *pollo asado* (broiled chicken).

New Mexican cuisine has many differences from Mexican and Tex-Mex cuisine. When you order chili (spelled *chile* in New Mexico), you typically get a red or green chile stew made without beans, although refried beans are usually served on the side. Sometimes, however, the red or green chile will contain wheat flour as a thickener. If it's pure chile, diced and cooked down, you can have it poured over a burger (sans bun), a steak, or a chicken breast.

Good rule of thumb: You'll do best with fajitas (without tortillas) and steaks (*carne asada*).

Hotel Restaurants**

Restaurants in hotels run the gamut from being little more than greasy spoons to serving healthy gourmet meals. One guiding rule in hotel restaurants is this: you almost always get what you pay for, which means you'll do better at more upscale hotel restaurants.

Upscale, of course, usually means more expensive. This isn't much of a problem if you're traveling on a business expense account. If you're on the road, however, and, like most people, have some financial constraints, consider staying at a less expensive hotel (or motel) but eating at restaurants where healthier foods are served. In smaller cities, ask about local restaurants.

The major hotel chains, such as Hilton and Marriott, almost always have a good restaurant on site, or the front desk can recommend nearby restaurants.

Good rule of thumb: Try salads, chicken, seafood, and meats.

What Should You Order to Drink?

It's important that you stop consuming soft drinks and alcohol. As substitutes, consider a glass of plain water with a wedge of lemon to enhance its taste or a glass of sparkling mineral water with a wedge of lime. As sparkling waters go, we favor the European brands, such as San Pellegrino, Gerolsteiner, Blu, and Perrier. They're also rich in calcium and magnesium, which are good for you.

Another option is iced tea—black, green, or herbal—as long as it contains no added sugar. Although black and green teas have caffeine, they also contain L-theanine, a naturally occurring chemical that has a calming effect. In addition, green tea inhibits alpha-glucosidase, an enzyme that breaks down sugar and starches in the digestive tract. Coffee, in small amounts (one or two cups daily), may reduce your long-term risk of developing diabetes, but much of the research on coffee is contradictory.

10

The Best Supplements for Improving Blood Sugar

Nutritional supplements can enhance the benefits that result from improved eating habits and can speed the healing process as you recover from prediabetes. Supplements contain concentrated amounts of vitamins, vitaminlike nutrients, minerals, or herbs and are sold in capsules, tablets, and sometimes liquids. They help in a variety of ways, such as by lowering blood sugar, improving insulin function, and reducing the risk of disease complications. Some supplements have very rapid and obvious effects, and others have more subtle benefits over the long term.

In this chapter, we explain why you should take supplements, and we describe those we have found to help prediabetes and diabetes. Certain supplements can reduce appetite and hunger and can promote weight loss, but they work by improving glucose tolerance, not by being "weight-loss pills" per se.

Do You Need Nutritional Supplements?

People sometimes ask us whether supplements are necessary. The sad fact is that nutritional deficiencies are commonplace in the United States, Europe, and Asia, a sign that it is difficult for people to obtain adequate or optimal levels of nutrients from food alone. The following

**Percentage of Americans Not Consuming
the Recommended Intakes of Nutrients**

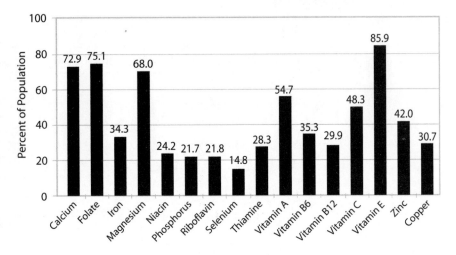

graph, compiled from U. S. Department of Agriculture nutrition data, shows the percentages of Americans who do not obtain the recommended amounts of many vitamins and minerals.

We believe that nutritional supplements are essential for health, especially for people who have prediabetes or weight problems. There are several reasons behind our thinking, which you may want to share with your own physician.

- People who are prediabetic or overweight have a history of eating nutrient-poor foods. (Otherwise, they would not have developed these diseases.) They consequently suffer from various nutritional deficiencies, which may range from marginal to very serious. These deficiencies impair the body's ability to regulate blood sugar and insulin, and they increase the risk of developing a wide range of health problems.

- Diabetes interferes with the activity of many nutrients, and prediabetes likely does as well. For example, people with diabetes do not efficiently convert beta-carotene, a beneficial antioxidant found in fruits and vegetables, to vitamin A. Low vitamin A levels result in night blindness, characterized by poor adjustment to darkness and bright lights. People with diabetes tend to have low levels of many nutrients, including vitamin C, vitamin D, and omega-3 fats.

• Excess body fat interferes with the normal distribution of nutrients in the body, often creating deficiencylike states. The reason is that fat cells serve as a nutrient sinkhole, in which many vitamins and minerals get deposited. When nutrients are stored in fat, they are withheld from other parts of the body, such as the liver, the heart, or the brain.

The Value of Nutrient Testing

Ideally, people should be tested to determine the nutrient levels in their bodies before they take high doses of individual supplements— that is, doses beyond those found in high-potency multivitamins. At the Center for the Improvement of Human Functioning International, a government-certified, on-site testing laboratory has measured people's nutrient levels for more than thirty years.

Each patient who comes to the center undergoes blood tests to assess his or her nutrient levels and also is given more conventional medical tests. This is a scientific approach, what some people call evidence-based medicine. Doctors at the center strive to correct nutrient deficiencies and imbalances that contribute to prediabetes, diabetes, overweight, and many other health problems. (In contrast, more conventional drug therapies tend to mask, but not correct, signs of vitamin and mineral deficiencies.) Following this approach, we treat patients appropriately, neither overtreating nor undertreating them.

Follow-up testing tracks changes in nutrient levels. These changes usually correlate with a reduction in physical symptoms and fewer laboratory markers of disease. After doing follow-up tests, we adjust patients' supplement programs to their changing needs.

Testing for nutrient levels is not as uncommon as you might think. The vast majority of doctors will test patients for potassium deficiency. For example, patients often tell their doctors about leg cramps and fatigue. If the doctor notices that the patient is taking a diuretic, he or she will suspect that the drug is depleting the patient's potassium reserves faster than his or her diet can replenish them. Most doctors will order a potassium level (often included in multiple-chemistry screening

QUICK TIP

Supplement-Drug Interactions

If you're taking any drug, including metformin or insulin, to control your blood sugar, you should be aware that either dietary improvements or nutritional supplements will likely lower your medication requirements. That's actually good because every physician knows patients are better off when they take less medicine.

Alpha-lipoic acid, R-lipoic acid, biotin, chromium, Pycnogenol, and silymarin can have a positive effect on blood sugar or insulin in a matter of weeks, especially if you combine two or more of these supplements. As a result, you may gradually begin to feel overmedicated and your blood sugar may dip too low. If you are taking a glucose-regulating or insulin-sensitizing drug, let your physician know and ask him or her to adjust the dose and the timing of your medications. Please do not make changes in your medication without consulting your physician.

panels) to confirm their hunch. If the patient's potassium is low, the doctor will typically prescribe a supplement in doses greater than the recommended daily allowance in order to correct the deficiency. Although potassium is indeed a nutrient, most doctors are not taught to think of it as such. Hence, they do not think that they are practicing nutritional medicine when they test for and treat potassium deficiency.

Of course, we realize that many people don't have the opportunity (or the money) to measure their nutrient levels. For this reason, we've organized our supplement recommendations for people who supplement without a physician's guidance, although we urge you to always inform your physician what you are doing. Many physicians do not have an in-depth understanding of nutritional therapies, and often patients must enlighten their doctors.

How Supplements Can Benefit You

Nutrients form the building blocks of the hundreds of thousands of bio-chemicals that are made within our bodies. Here are some reasons why nutritional supplements can help you to tackle prediabetes and your weight.

- Vitamins and minerals function as essential precursors and cofactors for all of the other biochemicals made by the body.

- Extra amounts of vitamins and minerals can strengthen weak or impaired biochemical pathways.

- Some vitamins and minerals can lower blood-sugar levels and enhance insulin function.

- Many vitamins and minerals improve liver function, which is important because this organ helps to regulate blood sugar and fats.

- Some nutrients can help to maintain normal muscle mass, which in turn aids in burning blood sugar.

- A few supplements can dampen appetite, leading to less eating and subsequent weight loss.

- Many people have above-average requirements for vitamins and minerals, for reasons relating to genetics or stress, and supplements can help to satisfy these greater needs.

How Should You Start Supplementing?

We recommend that you start with the basics—namely, multivitamin and multimineral supplements—to reduce your risk of having nutrient deficiencies. You should also have clear objectives when you move beyond multivitamins and multiminerals. For example, one might be to reduce your blood-sugar levels. Finally, remember that supplements work best if they accompany a healthy diet and are not used as an antidote for eating too many junk foods.

Creating a Sound Supplement Program

We would like you to take a high-potency multivitamin supplement as a foundation, which you can build on with other supplements. By "high potency," we mean a supplement containing 20 to 50 mg each of vitamins B1, B2, B3, and B6. (These amounts are much higher than the government's recommended daily amounts, but we believe those official amounts are unreasonably low.) If you get a supplement with 20 to 50 mg of these four nutrients, the relative dosages of other vitamins will usually fall into place.

We suggest buying supplements at health food or natural food stores because these products do not usually contain any sugar or artificial colors. (Supplements sold at pharmacies and discount stores often contain sugar, artificial colors, and cheaper, poorly absorbed ingredients.) You will also have a wide variety of excellent brands to choose from, including Carlson, Solgar, and many other companies. If you want to take a minimum of pills, we recommend that you take Carlson's Nutra-Support Diabetes, a multivitamin-multimineral that was formulated for people with prediabetes and diabetes. In addition to vitamins and minerals, it contains many vitaminlike substances that can help to maintain normal blood-sugar levels and insulin function.

In addition to a daily high-potency multivitamin, with dosages in the range listed in the following chart, we recommend that you take a separate multimineral supplement. Minerals are much bulkier than vitamins, and it's nearly impossible to get all of the minerals in their recommended amounts into a single tablet or capsule, especially when combined with vitamins. Depending on your specific health issues, you may want to build on this multimineral supplement with larger amounts of other supplements.

Vitamins

Vitamin A (not beta-carotene)	5,000 IU
Vitamin B1	20–50 mg
Vitamin B2	20–50 mg
Vitamin B3	20–75 mg
Vitamin B6	20–75 mg
Vitamin B12	70–500 mcg
Biotin	600–5,000 mcg
Choline	20–100 mg
Folic acid	400–800 mcg
Inositol	20–100 mg
Pantothenic acid	20–100 mg
Vitamin C	500–1,000 mg
Vitamin D	400–1,000 IU

| Vitamin E | 200–400 IU |
| Vitamin K | 50–100 mcg |

Minerals

Calcium	800–1,000 mg
Chromium	200–400 mcg
Copper	500 mcg to 1 mg
Iodine	50–150 mcg
Iron	0 mg
Manganese	5–10 mg
Magnesium	200–400 mg
Phosphorus	0 mg
Potassium	10–50 mg
Selenium	200 mcg
Zinc	15–30 mg

Be Cautious with Iron and Copper

Both iron and copper are essential nutrients, but they can be harmful in large amounts. We recommend that you *not* take a multimineral supplement that contains iron, unless you have been diagnosed as iron deficient. Considerable research indicates that high iron levels are strongly associated with the risk of developing diabetes and heart disease.

Although copper is not as problematic as iron, do pay close attention to the zinc-copper ratio. Many people with diabetes have high copper levels relative to zinc. To offset this problem, your multimineral supplement should have at least fifteen times more zinc than copper, unless your doctor has diagnosed you as copper deficient. If you take more than 25 mg of zinc daily, add 500 mcg to 1 mg of copper.

Your Next Step in Supplementing

The next step targets more specific health concerns, and we recommend that you take certain nutrients in amounts well above those found in almost all multivitamin and multimineral supplements.

Some supplements have multiple benefits, reflecting their diverse bio-chemical activities. If you want to take a particular supplement for more than one purpose, use the highest listed dosage, instead of adding together multiple dosages. For example, we recommend 1,000 mcg of chromium daily to improve insulin function and blood sugar, and we also recommend 500 mcg daily for depression. If you want to use chromium to address both health issues, stick to the higher dose of 1,000 mcg.

Our Top Supplement Choices

We don't expect you to take every supplement described in this chapter. For reversing prediabetes and controlling appetite and weight, however, we have six top choices. Your particular needs should determine which of these supplements you take.

1. *Alpha-lipoic acid* and *R-lipoic acid* improve insulin function and can lower blood sugar.
2. *Chromium* improves insulin function and lowers blood sugar.
3. *Biotin* plays a crucial role in managing insulin and blood sugar.
4. *Omega-3 fish oils* lower triglyceride levels and may help in weight reduction.
5. *Vitamin C* combats fatigue, a common symptom in prediabetes and overweight, and it might also help to burn fat.
6. *Pycnogenol*, a powerful natural antioxidant, may lower blood sugar, reduce inflammation, and improve many complications of diabetes.

Supplements That Help to Reduce Your Appetite (and Maybe Control Weight)

Several supplements may help you to lose weight by decreasing your appetite. These supplements are most effective when you use them in conjunction with the protein- and vegetable-rich eating habits described in earlier chapters.

- *Alpha-lipoic acid.* This antioxidant has been sold in Europe for decades as a prescription drug for the treatment of diabetes and diabetes-related nerve pain and numbness. In animal experiments, researchers found that alpha-lipoic acid reduced appetite, sped up metabolism (that is, the ability to burn calories), and promoted weight loss. It works at least in part by suppressing an enzyme that stimulates appetite and hunger. Try 100 mg a few minutes before each meal.

- *R-lipoic acid.* This type of lipoic acid is chemically identical to the one found in nature, and it accounts for half of the alpha-lipoic acid molecule. R-lipoic acid is more expensive than alpha-lipoic acid, but it has more biological activity. As an alternative to alpha-lipoic acid, try 100 mg a few minutes before meals.

- *Chromium.* Chromium is an essential mineral that plays a central role in normal insulin function and the burning of blood sugar. The two leading forms of this mineral are chromium polynicotinate and chromium picolinate, and both forms have been extensively tested in people. It's often difficult to sort through the competitive claims and counterclaims for these products; however, we are impressed by the research of Harry Preuss, M.D., of Georgetown University, who found that the chromium polynicotinate form promotes fat loss but preserves muscle. Some research also suggests that chromium polynicotinate is better absorbed than other forms. (The term *polynicotinate* indicates that the chromium is bound to vitamin B3, sometimes called nicotinic acid.)

  Meanwhile, research has shown that chromium picolinate helps to prevent weight gain associated with the use of the diabetic drug glipizide (Glucotrol). Other forms of chromium, such as chromium glycinate chelate, may work as well. Regardless of the specific form, the research on chromium and diabetes points to the greater efficacy of higher dosages, so we recommend trying 500 mcg twice daily. Another product, Super CitriMax, combines chromium polynicotinate with calcium and potassium hydroxycitrates, which together seem to reduce appetite and may help with weight loss.

- *Omega-3 fish oils.* People with prediabetes and diabetes almost always have low levels of the omega-3 fats. Omega-3 fish oil supplements improve glucose tolerance, and some research suggests that they may help the body to burn fat. In recent animal experiments, docosahexaenoic acid (DHA), one of the key omega-3 fats, blocked the formation of fat cells while promoting the breakdown of existing fat cells. Try 1,000 to 3,000 mg daily of omega-3 fish oils or 500 to 1,000 mg daily of DHA.

- *Vitamin C.* People need this vitamin to make carnitine, a substance that helps to transport fat into cells, where it is burned for energy. Without enough vitamin C, carnitine production slows. One of the most common signs of low vitamin C intake is fatigue, mainly because the body cannot make enough carnitine. Take at least 1,000 mg of vitamin C daily.

- *Pycnogenol.* This complex of antioxidants, extracted from the bark of French maritime pine trees, inhibits the activity of alpha-glucosidase, one of the enzymes that breaks down sugar and carbohydrates during digestion. The mechanism is similar to the diabetes drug acarbose, but research has found that Pycnogenol is 190 times more active than acarbose in inhibiting alpha-glucosidase. As a result, some carbs pass through the gut without being broken down into glucose or stored as fat. Being a natural substance, Pycnogenol is also much safer than acarbose.

- *PGX.* Known more technically as PolyGlycopleX, this is a particularly good dietary fiber supplement sold by Natural Factors as SlimStyles granules and capsules. Taken just a few minutes before meals, it reduces appetite. Studies have shown that after three weeks of supplementation, PGX significantly lowers blood-sugar and insulin levels. Although the label suggests weight-loss benefits, we think that any weight loss results from improved blood-sugar and insulin levels.

- *Phase 2 Starch Neutralizer.* Although we have some reservations about starch-blocking supplements, this particular brand has some scientific support for inhibiting the activity of alpha amylase, one of the gut's starch-digesting enzymes. By blocking the activity of alpha amylase, Phase 2 prevents the absorption of some carbohydrates. We think it's important to limit the consumption of refined carbohy-drates (including sugars), but some people might benefit from sup-plements. Still, Phase 2 and similar supplements are not a substitute for better eating habits.

Top Supplements That Lower Blood Sugar and Improve Insulin Function

These supplements have been shown to reduce blood-sugar levels, improve insulin function, or do both. Most of the studies used only the supplements, not dietary changes; however, combining these supple-ments with improved eating habits will greatly enhance their benefits. *Note*: If you combine two or more of some of the following supple-ments—specifically, alpha-lipoic acid or R-lipoic acid, chromium pico-linate, silymarin, American ginseng, or glycine—you may be able to reduce their dosages by 25 to 50 percent.

- *Alpha-lipoic acid.* This antioxidant actually works through a variety of biochemical pathways, and people who faithfully take it often ben-efit from an improvement in insulin function and a gradual decrease in blood-sugar levels. If you are prediabetic, take 100 mg fifteen minutes before each meal; if you are diabetic, take 200 mg before each meal. Do not take more than 600 mg daily.

- *R-lipoic acid.* This form of lipoic acid may actually yield greater ben-efits than alpha-lipoic acid in lowering blood sugar and improving insulin activity. The problem is that it is considerably more expensive than alpha-lipoic acid (which contains 50 percent of the R-lipoic form). Take 100 to 200 mg a few minutes before each meal.

- *Chromium.* Symptoms of chromium deficiency—increased glucose, insulin, total cholesterol, and triglycerides—resemble those of predi-abetes. This certainly doesn't mean that chromium alone will reverse prediabetes; however, many studies have shown that either chromium polynicotinate or chromium picolinate supplements do in fact improve insulin function and can lead to improved glucose tolerance. Based on the research, the most effective dose of chromium appears to be 1,000 mcg, or 500 mcg twice daily with meals. We recommend the chromium polynicotinate form, also called niacin-bound chromium, which has a strong record of safety and use in supplements, beverages, and foods.

- *Biotin.* This little known B-complex vitamin is essential for the manufacture of insulin, and it also has insulinlike activity. Biotin regulates genes involved in the metabolism of glucose, amino acids, and fatty acids. Some supplements combine biotin with either chromium or R-lipoic acid. Although the official recommended amount is only 30 mcg daily, much larger (and safe) dosages have been found helpful in diabetes. Try 500 to 1,000 mcg two or three times daily with meals.

- *Pycnogenol.* This antioxidant can lead to impressive reductions in fasting blood sugar and postmeal increases in blood sugar. In one study, people with diabetes took 50 mg of Pycnogenol daily for three weeks and benefited from an average 10 percent decrease in fasting blood-sugar levels; however, the benefits increased with larger amounts of Pycnogenol. Taking dosages ranging from 100 to 200 mg daily for three weeks resulted in almost a 13 percent reduction in fasting blood sugar. Over several months, these high dosages of Pycnogenol led to an 8.1 percent reduction in HbA_{1c} levels.

- *Silymarin.* This extract of the herb milk thistle (*Silybum marianum*) is a potent antioxidant and is widely used to enhance liver function. That's important because the liver works in tandem with the pancreas to regulate glucose levels. In a year-long study, 600 mg daily of silymarin reduced blood-sugar levels in seriously ill diabetic patients by 9.5 to 15 percent. The patients also benefited from lower levels of sugar in the urine, lower HbA_{1c} levels, and lower insulin requirements. Other studies have found similar benefits. For prediabetes, we recommend 100 mg with meals two or three times daily.

- *Vitamin D.* In recent years, vitamin D deficiencies have commonly been found in the general population. People who are overweight or those with diabetes are especially susceptible to vitamin D deficiency. In a large study, almost two of every three people with diabetes were deficient in vitamin D. In another study, 15 percent of obese patients were deficient in vitamin D. The reason, according to Anastassios G. Pittas, M.D., of the Tufts-New England Medical Center, is that vitamin D is stored in fat cells, away from other tissues that need it. A three-year study by Pittas found that taking 700 IU of vitamin D, plus 500 mg of calcium, led to smaller increases in fasting blood sugar, compared with people given placebos. We suspect most of the benefits were related to the extra vitamin D, not to the calcium.

For years, people were warned that large amounts of vitamin D were toxic. It turns out that all those fears go back to a 1984 study of six patients in India, and no one ever bothered to measure their vitamin D levels. If you stand in the summer sun, your body will make about 10,000 IU of vitamin D in fifteen minutes. Current recommendations from researchers at Harvard University and the Boston University Medical School are 1,000 to 2,000 IU daily, and many people can benefit from 4,000 to 10,000 IU daily without any risk of harm. Carlson Laboratories is one of the few companies that sells 1,000, 2,000 and 4,000 IU capsules of vitamin D. We recommend 1,000 to 2,000 IU of vitamin D daily, and a little more if you have dark skin.

Some Other Supplements That Might Also Help to Lower Blood Sugar

- *Glycine.* Research dating back to 1932 has shown that large supplemental dosages of glycine, a building block of protein, can reduce blood-sugar levels in both healthy and diabetic subjects. It works by accelerating the burning of blood sugar. In one study, Mary C. Gannon, Ph.D., and her colleagues at the University of Minnesota, Minneapolis, found that 3.6 to 5.4 grams of glycine reduced postmeal elevations in blood sugar by 15 percent. Try 2 grams of glycine with meals and in combination with any of the other recommended supplements.

- *American ginseng.* Several studies have found that American ginseng (also called *Panax ginseng* and *Panax quinquefolius*) can significantly lower blood sugar in both healthy and diabetic subjects. Researchers at the University of Toronto found that 3 to 9 grams of ginseng reduced blood-sugar levels by 20 to 38 percent after a glucose-tolerance test. Similar reductions in blood sugar are likely after meals. Because the difference between the doses wasn't significant, save yourself some money and stick with the lower dose. Try 3 grams daily.

- *N-acetylcysteine (NAC)*. This potent antioxidant may be of particular benefit in polycystic ovary syndrome (PCOS), a condition that involves insulin resistance, elevated testosterone levels, and infertility. In one study, researchers asked twenty women with PCOS to take 600 mg of NAC three times daily for four weeks. By the end of the study, the women's insulin levels had decreased by one-third, and their testosterone levels dropped by more than half. NAC may have more general benefits in preventing insulin resistance, especially for people who eat a high-fructose diet. Take 1,000 to 2,000 IU daily. *Note*: Because of its high sulfur content, NAC may smell like rotten eggs.

- *Magnesium*. People with diabetes are commonly deficient in magnesium, a mineral that is directly and indirectly involved in managing blood-sugar levels. In an analysis of nine well-controlled clinical trials, researchers concluded that magnesium supplements could significantly lower fasting blood sugar and raise the "good" high-density lipoprotein form of cholesterol. We recommend taking either magnesium citrate or magnesium aspartate, 200 mg twice a day with meals. If you take too much, you will develop loose stools.

- *Vanadium*. Although vanadium is not (yet) considered an essential nutrient for people, it does appear to have a role in normal glucose tolerance. Vanadium is an insulin mimic, meaning that it works like insulin to help cells absorb and burn blood sugar. Animal studies have found that vanadium can lower fasting glucose, LDL cholesterol, triglyceride levels, and blood pressure. Several human studies, with very large doses of vanadium, show promising results. The downside is that vanadium, in large doses, may contribute to depression and kidney problems. For this reason, we recommend that supplements, typically in the form of vanadyl sulfate, be used cautiously or under your physician's guidance. If you're taking it on your own, dosages of vanadyl sulfate up to 1 mg (1,000 mcg) daily should be completely safe. Your physician may recommend 5 to 25 mg daily.

- *Iodine*. The official recommended daily amount of iodine is a miniscule 150 mcg, compared with an estimated daily dietary intake of 13.8 mg in Japan (which is almost a hundred times higher!). Because soil

SPECIFIC BRANDS OF SUPPLEMENTS WE LIKE

Trying to remember the large number of nutritional supplements, along with all sorts of health claims, can make shopping confusing. Based on our experiences, we like and recommend the following specific products.

- *Carlson Nutra-Support Diabetes.* This high-potency multivitamin was formulated to enhance the nutrition of people who have prediabetes and diabetes. If you want to keep your tablets and capsules to an absolute minimum, this is the one product you should take. More information is available at www.carlsonlabs.com.

- *Carlson Cod Liver Oil.* Of the many fish and cod-liver oil products on the market, this is one of the best. It provides the omega-3 fats and vitamin D. It's a liquid with a light lemon taste. More information is available at www.carlsonlabs.com.

- *Chromate.* Many companies sell Chromate, the patented brand of chromium polynicotinate (niacin-bound chromium). Research shows that it helps to burn fat while preserving muscle. More information is available at www.interhealthusa.com.

- *Pycnogenol.* You can buy this antioxidant complex from a great number of companies. It has multiple benefits for people who have prediabetes and diabetes, including improvements in blood sugar and diabetes-related eye disease and skin ulcers. It also lessens a variety of cardiovascular risk factors. More information is available at www.pycnogenol.com.

- *Insulow.* This product combines R-lipoic acid with biotin, two important nutrients for controlling and reversing prediabetes. More information is available at www.insulow.com.

- *SuperCitrimax.* We're generally wary of products that claim to lower appetite, burn fat, and promote weight loss. Super CitriMax is built around chromium polynicotinate, and it works in large part by improving insulin function and glucose control. More information is available at www.supercitrimax.com.

- *Diachrome.* This supplement combines chromium picolinate with biotin. More information is available at www.diachrome.com.

and water levels of iodine are low in many parts of the United States, including vast parts of the Midwest, for years commercial salt has been iodized to prevent gross deficiencies. Large amounts of iodine, however, may be beneficial.

Jorge D. Flechas, M.D., of Hendersonville, North Carolina, has reported that large doses of iodine are especially helpful for people with diabetes. He has found that supplemental high-dose iodine leads to a normalization of HbA_{1c} and blood-sugar levels, and some patients also lose substantial amounts of weight. Flechas has used 50 to 100 mg of iodine, but the need for such high doses is best determined by a nutritionally oriented physician. In these circumstances, Iodoral (sold only to physicians) is the iodine supplement of choice. It contains 5 mg of iodine and 7.5 mg of potassium iodide, approximating the daily Japanese consumption. Because large amounts of iodine increase the activity of the thyroid gland, prompting it to produce more hormones, we recommend that you work with a nutritionally oriented physician who starts with an iodine/urine loading test.

Supplements That Help You to Maintain Muscle

Muscle cells do the best job of burning blood sugar and fat for energy. Some nutrients, particularly vitamin D and leucine, help to maintain normal muscle mass. This is especially important if you are sedentary, overweight, or elderly.

- *Vitamin D.* Short of regular exercise, vitamin D supplements may be one of the best ways to maintain normal muscle mass. Your body needs vitamin D to make protein and to produce muscle cells. Taking vitamin D supplements won't give you the muscles of Arnold Schwarzenegger, but they will help you hold your own against the age-related decline in muscle tissue, which increases your susceptibility to developing prediabetes. Vitamin D will also reduce your risk of falling, which can lead to broken bones. Take 1,000 to 2,000 IU daily.
- *Leucine.* This amino acid, or protein building block, plays a particularly important role in maintaining muscle mass. If you eat substantial amounts of animal protein, you probably get enough leucine.

Adding a little supplemental leucine, however, may slow the age-related decline in muscle mass. In a recent study, the addition of supplemental leucine helped seniors to synthesize as much muscle as young men do.

Supplements That Help You Deal with Diabetic Complications

Some supplements may be helpful adjuncts to other nutritional and medical therapies for relieving or lessening the risk of developing diabetic complications. These are very serious conditions, so please work with your physician in treating them.

- *Neuropathy.* Neuropathy is a general term that refers to nerve damage, which may be characterized by extreme sensitivity to pain or numbness. Alpha-lipoic acid is the number-one choice for treating neuropathy. Try 200 mg three times daily. In addition, gamma-linolenic acid, part of a family of essential dietary fats, can also help with diabetes-related nerve damage. Try 100 mg twice daily in combination with alpha-lipoic acid.

- *Eye disease.* Diabetes increases the risk of developing virtually all serious eye diseases. Inadequate intake of vitamin A, which is characterized by night blindness (i.e., difficulty seeing in the dark or adjusting to bright lights), is also associated with serious eye diseases. Take 25,000 IU of vitamin A (not beta-carotene) daily for thirty days, then reduce the dosage to 10,000 IU daily. If, however, you are a woman of childbearing age and there is any chance that you might get pregnant, do not take more than 5,000 IU daily.

    To reduce your long-term risk of developing macular degeneration and cataracts, take 5 mg daily of lutein, either as lutein esters or unbound (free) lutein. For active retinal eye disease, try 15 to 30 mg daily of either lutein esters or unbound lutein. In addition, Pycnogenol, 100 to 150 mg twice daily, may be helpful in treating diabetes-related retinopathy.

- *Kidney disease.* High blood-sugar levels are toxic to the kidneys. N-acetylcysteine can often restore normal kidney function, if the damage is not too severe. Take 500 mg three times daily.

- *Poor circulation.* Reduced circulation and fragile blood vessels are commonly associated with prediabetes and diabetes. The reduced circulation is a consequence of endothelial dysfunction—essentially, an abnormal stiffening of blood vessels. Fragile blood vessels can lead to bruising, edema (fluid retention), and inflammation. Several supplements are extremely helpful for circulation: vitamin E, 200 to 400 IU daily; vitamin C, 1,000 to 3,000 mg daily; Pycnogenol, 150 to 200 mg daily; and L-arginine, 1,000 mg twice daily.

- *Hypertension.* Elevated blood pressure is almost always related to high insulin levels. Several supplements can enhance dietary changes and lower your blood pressure. Sustained release L-arginine is the precursor to a natural compound that relaxes blood vessels. We recommend 1,000 mg twice daily of Perfusia-SR, from Thorne Research. Check with your doctor if you take medications to control your blood pressure. In addition, you might also try 10 mg daily of lycopene and 100 mg daily of Pycnogenol.

11

Overcome Related Health Problems

I magine, for a moment, that prediabetes and overweight form the thick trunk of a tree. The trunk grows into limbs, which you can envision as the major health consequences of having prediabetes and being overweight. These limbs, in turn, branch out and lead to many more health problems.

So many of today's ailments, from purely physical illnesses to mood disorders, are intertwined with prediabetes and overweight. Even when prediabetes and overweight are not the direct causes of health problems, they exacerbate the symptoms, the complications, and the progression of diseases. Trimming the branches, so to speak, such as by prescribing drugs, may improve some of the symptoms, but it does not change the underlying disease processes—the root of the problem.

In this chapter, we focus on some of the limbs and branches, that is, the common health consequences of prediabetes, diabetes, and overweight. We touched on a few of these issues briefly in chapter 1, but it is important that we revisit some in greater detail. As you read the following sections, you'll notice that many of these health problems overlap. That's because they have similar roots in eating habits, prediabetes, and overweight.

As you follow our dietary recommendations, many of these health concerns will self-correct—an experience we call "side benefits." Yet some people will have more of an uphill climb than others do in dealing with their prediabetes and weight. Even if you never achieve absolutely perfect blood-sugar levels or a normal weight, you will be far better off than if you had done nothing.

Premature Aging, Diabetes, and Overweight

Do you often feel older than you should? If you have prediabetes or diabetes or are overweight, you are in fact aging faster than a healthy person your age does.

Glucose tolerance decreases with age, even in healthy people, as part of the biological breakdown and inefficiency that come with growing older. Researchers have long viewed diabetes as a unique window to the aging process. With accelerated aging, bodies break down sooner than they would otherwise, resulting in many different symptoms and the early onset of various diseases.

What are the exact links between diabetes and aging? First, high blood-sugar levels trigger a biological chain reaction that leads to the increased production of free radicals. These destructive molecules damage genes, cell proteins, and membranes, diminishing cell function throughout your body. For more than fifty years, we have known that free radicals contribute to aging and disease, and high levels of free radicals are also associated with most complications of diabetes.

Second, elevated blood-sugar levels generate large numbers of "advanced glycation end products," or glycotoxins, in which sugars fuse with proteins and render the proteins virtually useless. This is significant because, on a biochemical level, proteins are the workhorses of the body. Advanced glycation end products also damage the genetic code in your body's cells. The HbA_{1c} test, described in chapter 1, measures glycation damage.

Third, high levels of insulin increase the risk of two age-related causes of death: heart disease and cancer. Type 2 diabetics who receive insulin injections to control their blood sugar are more likely to suffer heart attacks, compared with people who do not get insulin injections. In a very real sense, insulin is both a growth and an aging hormone, essential to life in small amounts but harmful in excess.

Insulin also encourages the proliferation of cells, a process needed for normal growth and healing but also for the growth of cancers. High insulin levels are strongly associated with many different types of cancer, including cancers of the breast, the prostate, and the colon. In a nutshell, excess insulin increases a person's odds of dying at any age, whether from diabetes, heart disease, or cancer.

Heart and Circulatory Problems, Blood Sugar, and Insulin

People with diabetes are four times more likely to have heart attacks than are people who don't have diabetes. What is the risk if you are pre-diabetic? It turns out that slight increases in blood sugar, even when they're still in the normal range, substantially increase your risk of having a heart attack. High levels of insulin, cholesterol and triglycerides, along with markers of inflammation and clotting, further boost your odds of having a heart attack.

All of these cardiovascular risk factors stem from the same eating habits that cause prediabetes and overweight. Elevations in total cholesterol, low-density lipoprotein (LDL) cholesterol, very low-density lipoprotein (VLDL) cholesterol, and triglycerides almost always improve when people start to eat lean proteins (which are low in saturated fat), fish, and vegetables and avoid processed and other junk foods. In fact, eating more coldwater fish, rich in the omega-3 fats, can significantly reduce the amount of small LDL particles, the most dangerous kind. Supplements of omega-3 fish oils will have a similar benefit.

Cardiovascular disease develops through a variety of mechanisms, not just because of high blood fats. For example, a low intake of vitamins B6, B12, and folic acid raises high blood concentrations of homocysteine, a substance that damages blood vessel walls. This blood vessel damage invites cholesterol deposits as the body makes a misguided attempt to heal itself. Taking these B vitamins lowers homocysteine levels and protects blood vessels.

Endothelial dysfunction is another risk factor for diabetes and coronary heart disease, although it is not routinely measured. The endothelium is a thin layer of cells lining the inside of blood vessels. In healthy people, it flexes a little like an undulating snake and helps the heart to circulate blood. In endothelial dysfunction, blood vessels stiffen and become inflexible, circulation decreases, and blood pressure increases to compensate. Eating foods that are high in sugar, refined carbohydrates, and trans fats induces endothelial dysfunction within minutes, and endothelial dysfunction is common in people with prediabetes, diabetes, and weight problems.

Inflammation is now regarded as the fundamental cause of coronary heart (artery) disease. Chronic low-grade inflammation damages the heart's major blood vessel walls, and the body deposits cholesterol in an effort to protect the arteries. Sustained inflammation weakens the cholesterol deposits, making them more likely to rupture and cause deadly clots in smaller blood vessels. Low-grade inflammation is easily measured with the high-sensitivity C-reactive protein test, and diets rich in sugar and other refined carbohydrates are strongly associated with elevated C-reactive protein levels. High levels of C-reactive protein are common in people who are diabetic or overweight.

Similarly, an abnormal tendency toward coagulation—that is, blood clotting—is commonly found in people with prediabetes and diabetes, and it is also a risk factor for developing heart disease. Doctors can measure clotting speeds through a variety of tests. High levels of fibrinogen, one of the clotting compounds, points to a greater tendency toward clots developing within blood vessels.

If you follow our dietary recommendations for eating fish, lean meats, and high-fiber vegetables, your total cholesterol, LDL cholesterol, and triglycerides will likely decrease. These same eating habits will reduce inflammation and clotting to more normal levels. You can enhance the benefits by adding various dietary supplements, some of which we discussed in earlier chapters.

Supplements That Might Reduce Your Cardiovascular Risk

To lower your cholesterol and LDL cholesterol, consider taking one or two of these supplements:

- *Beta-sitosterol*, 1.3 to 3.6 grams daily. This is a natural compound, also referred to as phytosterols, found in vegetables. It reduces the absorption of cholesterol in the intestine.

- *Niacin*, 500 to 1,000 mg daily. In addition to lowering total cholesterol and LDL cholesterol, this particular form of vitamin B3 raises the "good" high-density lipoprotein form of cholesterol. *Note*: Taking niacin causes a flushing sensation, in which you will turn beet red for about one hour. Some people find the reaction very uncomfortable, although it does ease with daily use.

- *Sytrinol*, 150 mg, once or twice daily. This supplement is a proprietary combination of beta-sitosterol, flavonoids, and tocotrienols (part of the vitamin E family of molecules).

- *Magnesium*, 300 to 400 mg daily. Inadequate levels of this mineral may increase your cholesterol levels.

- *Pantethine*, a form of the B-vitamin pantothenic acid, may also reduce cholesterol levels. Try 200 to 300 mg, three times daily.

To lower your triglycerides, take this supplement:

- *Omega-3 fish oils*, 1,000 to 3,000 mg daily. The omega-3s are the best supplement for lowering triglyceride levels.

To improve your endothelial function, take these supplements:

- *L-arginine*, 1,000 mg twice daily. This constituent of protein is the precursor to nitric oxide, the chemical that regulates blood vessel tone. The sustained-release type (called Profusia SR and made by Thorne Research) is longer acting.

- *Vitamin C*, 1,000 mg daily. This vitamin helps to maintain normal blood-vessel flexibility.

- *Vitamin E*, 400 IU of the natural "d-alpha" form. Vitamin E helps to maintain blood vessel flexibility, and a combination of vitamins E and C is particularly beneficial. Vitamin E also prevents the free-radical oxidation of LDL cholesterol, a very early step in the development of heart disease.

- *Pycnogenol*, 100 to 200 mg daily. This remarkable antioxidant can improve endothelial function, particularly when combined with L-arginine.

To reduce inflammation, take these supplements:

- *Omega-3 fish oils*, 1,000 to 3,000 mg daily.
- *Pycnogenol*, 200 to 300 mg daily.
- *Vitamin E*, 400 IU daily of the natural form.
- *Ginger*, follow label directions (or make ginger tea).
- *Curcumin*, follow label directions.

To reduce clotting time, take these supplements:

- *Vitamin E*, 400 IU daily of the natural form.
- *Omega-3 fish oils*, 1,000 to 3,000 mg daily.
- *Garlic*, follow label directions (or eat one raw clove daily).

Erectile Dysfunction and Infertility in Men

Psychological issues can certainly impact a man's ability to have an erection, but most experts now believe that erectile dysfunction is primarily a vascular problem. In fact, doctors often interpret erectile dysfunction as a sign of cardiovascular disease, prediabetes, and diabetes. That's because the same nutritional and biochemical problems that cause endothelial dysfunction also lead to erectile dysfunction.

To form an erection, blood vessels in the penis must dilate and fill with blood. This ability of blood vessels to dilate depends on the activity of nitric oxide, a molecule that regulates blood vessel tone. The body makes nitric oxide from L-arginine, a constituent of protein. The conversion of L-arginine to nitric oxide requires the enzyme nitric oxide synthase, which depends on vitamin C.

Erectile dysfunction is a common problem in men who are either diabetic or overweight. Obese men have about twice the risk of suffering from erectile dysfunction, compared with men of normal weight. Again, eating too many foods that are high in sugar, refined carbohydrates, and trans fats interferes with endothelial function and leads to erectile dysfunction. In addition, smoking increases the risk of developing erectile dysfunction by 50 percent.

Men who are prediabetic and overweight tend to have low levels of testosterone, which would result in a low sex drive. A study by Finnish researchers found that an extra twenty pounds of weight decreased male fertility—the ability to make a woman pregnant—by 10 percent. If you see yourself in this description, ask your physician to measure your testosterone levels. If they are low—and only if they are low—ask him or her about taking supplemental DHEA (dehydroepiandrosterone).

HANK'S STORY
A Natural Solution for Erectile Dysfunction

At age thirty-eight, Hank was chubby and had moderately elevated blood sugar and high levels of triglycerides. These were early signs of prediabetes, but in other respects Hank seemed in fairly good health. His main complaint was about difficulty in forming and maintaining an erection. Both he and his wife were frustrated by their lack of sexual intimacy over the last couple of years.

Hank could have simply taken one of the popular drugs used to treat erectile dysfunction, but he had a personal aversion to drugs unless he felt them to be absolutely necessary. Erectile dysfunction is a common consequence of prediabetes and diabetes, so it was important to improve his blood sugar.

He adopted an eating plan that was rich in lean proteins and vegetables. He agreed to a fairly simple supplement regimen: a high-potency multivitamin, plus supplements of L-arginine and L-carnitine (both components of protein). L-arginine is essential for normal blood vessel and erectile function, and L-carnitine can also help in some cases of erectile dysfunction. During the next two months, Hank lost fifteen pounds, and his blood sugar and triglycerides decreased. He and his wife also began having sexual intercourse again.

Supplements That Might Help with Erectile Dysfunction

- *L-arginine*, 1,000 mg twice daily. Supplemental L-arginine can often restore normal endothelial function and can also have remarkable effects on erectile function. Of the many L-arginine supplements on the market, we recommend Profusia SR, made by Thorne Research. (See the resources for ordering information.) Take one capsule (1,000 mg) twice daily, at least one hour before or after eating any food. You can take the last dose, or an extra dose, about thirty to sixty minutes before intercourse, as long as you are otherwise healthy enough to be sexually active.

- *Pycnogenol*, 100 mg twice daily. The antioxidants in Pycnogenol may enhance the benefits of L-arginine.
- *Vitamin C*, 500 mg to 1,000 mg daily. Vitamin C enhances the activity of L-arginine.
- *L-carnitine*, 1,000 to 3,000 mg daily. This component of protein appears to work better than testosterone in the treatment of erectile dysfunction and, unlike the hormone, L-carnitine does not increase prostate size.

Cancer Risk, Insulin, and Blood Sugar

Being prediabetic, diabetic, or overweight substantially increases your risk of developing many different types of cancer. Much of this increased risk seems to be directly related to elevated insulin levels.

Insulin is an anabolic hormone, meaning that it promotes the growth of new cells. A little insulin is essential for life, but too much can fuel the growth of cancers. Meanwhile, high levels of glucose generate large numbers of destructive free radicals, which can damage the genetic code of cells and can create abnormal cells.

Overall, people with diabetes are about 25 percent more likely to develop cancer than are people who do not have diabetes. This greater risk applies mostly to cancers of the cervix, the colon and rectum, the endometrium, the esophagus, the kidneys, the liver, the pancreas, and the stomach. The odds of developing cancer of the liver and the pancreas, the two organs most involved in regulating insulin and blood sugar, are also especially high among people with diabetes.

Obesity accounts for more than a hundred thousand new cases of cancer each year in the United States. Obesity increases a person's risk of developing breast, colon, endometrial, kidney, esophageal, and pancreatic cancer, as well as non-Hodgkin's lymphoma and multiple myelomas. Being overweight also increases a woman's odds of dying from cancer, particularly ovarian cancer.

Prediabetes (usually diagnosed as insulin resistance) is common in patients with cancer. It may have contributed to the risk of cancer, and it may also be a consequence of metabolic changes from having cancer.

Supplements That Might Help to Reduce Your Cancer Risk

Eating a lot of fruits and vegetables reduces your risk of developing most cancers. Several individual supplements may also lessen your long-term risk of getting cancer.

- *Selenium*, 200 mcg daily
- *Vitamin E*, 400 IU daily, of the natural "d-alpha" form
- *Vitamin C*, 1,000 mg daily
- *N-acetylcysteine*, 500 to 1,000 mg daily

Polycystic Ovary Syndrome and Infertility in Women

Polycystic ovary syndrome (PCOS) is one of the most common causes of infertility. It may affect up to 10 percent of women of childbearing age, and the condition's three key diagnostic criteria are multiple ovarian cysts, excess production of testosterone (primarily a male hormone), and elevated levels of insulin.

The high levels of insulin, of course, point to insulin resistance, prediabetes, and sometimes diabetes. Other common symptoms of PCOS include overweight, facial hair, thinning of hair on the scalp, irregular menstrual periods, high blood pressure, acne, sleep apnea, endothelial dysfunction, and low-grade inflammation.

The treatment of PCOS focuses on improving insulin function and weight loss. Although some doctors favor the use of insulin-sensitizing drugs, dietary therapies can have great success. Tackle PCOS as you would prediabetes: emphasize eating lean proteins and vegetables, avoid all refined sugar and carbohydrates, and limit all other types of carbohydrates.

Supplements That Might Help to Reduce Your PCOS Risk

- *N-acetylcysteine*, 600 mg three times daily. In a study of women with PCOS, this dose of N-acetylcysteine led to significant decreases in testosterone and insulin. Testosterone levels dropped by more than half and insulin levels declined by about one-third in four weeks.

Several supplements known to improve glucose tolerance may also be helpful for PCOS. These supplements include the following.

- *Alpha-lipoic acid* or *R-lipoic acid*, 200 mg three times daily.
- *Chromium polynicotinate*, 400 to 1,000 mcg daily.
- *Silymarin*, 200 mg three times daily.

Stress, Prediabetes, and Overweight

Do you often feel stressed? If you do, you are more likely to become prediabetic. In one study, conducted at University College, London, researchers found that people who regularly experienced work-related stress over a period of fourteen years were twice as likely to become prediabetic.

When people feel stressed, their eating habits slide and they are more likely to eat fast foods and sugary junk foods. In addition, the sugar- and carb-rich foods that predispose a person toward developing prediabetes and becoming overweight are typically low in B vitamins. Low levels of these vitamins, particularly vitamin B1, interfere with carbohydrate metabolism. Sugary and high-carb foods also shortchange the brain of building blocks to make calming, stress-buffering nutrients.

An increase in cortisol, the body's main stress hormone, tends to occur in tandem with a rise in insulin. For example, a lack of sleep boosts cortisol levels that, along with insulin, promote the formation of belly fat. Furthermore, as cortisol levels go up, the hormone DHEA (dehydroepiandrosterone) tends to go down. DHEA, often considered an anti-aging hormone, is a precursor to our steroid hormones (including testosterone and estrogen), which decline with age.

Supplements That Might Help You to Reduce Stress

In addition to a diet of high-quality protein and high-fiber vegetables, consider trying these supplements.

- *B-complex vitamins*, high-potency formula (with dosages comparable to those described in chapter 10). Many of the B vitamins are necessary to make calming neurotransmitters—hence, their reputation as antistress nutrients.

- *Gamma-linolenic acid (GLA)*, 100 to 200 mg daily. This plant oil enhances the anti-inflammatory benefits of omega-3 fish oils. It also seems to moderate stress reactions.

- *Gamma-aminobutyric acid (GABA)* and *L-theanine*. These two amino acids (protein building blocks) work together to raise brain levels of GABA and take the edge off anxiety. Try 200 mg of GABA and 100 of L-theanine once or twice daily. The most reliable L-theanine brand is Suntheanine. Two excellent products containing L-theanine and GABA are Carlson's Mellow Mood and Allergy Research Group's 200 mg of Zen.

- *Lactium*, 200 mg daily. This supplement contains a proteinlike extract from dairy products that can ease stress-related anxiety.

Sleep Disorders, Overweight, and Prediabetes

Do you have trouble sleeping? An estimated 50 to 70 million Americans have chronic sleep disorders. Of that number, 18 million suffer specifically from sleep apnea, which impairs breathing. Many people with sleep apnea repeatedly wake up in the middle of the night and, because of interrupted sleep, have slower reflexes, poorer memory, and disjointed thinking the next day.

Inadequate sleep and a lack of quality sleep are strongly associated with prediabetes and diabetes. Researchers at the Boston University School of Medicine found that people who slept less than six hours or more than nine hours nightly were more likely to have glucose-tolerance problems, compared with people who got about eight hours of sleep. Other research has shown that a lack of sleep and of *quality* sleep increase blood-sugar levels and the risk of developing more severe diabetes.

In one study, published in the *Archives of Internal Medicine*, researchers found that overweight people slept almost two hours less a week than did people of normal weight. In other research, described at a meeting of the American Thoracic Society, women who slept only six hours nightly had a one-in-eight chance of being overweight, compared with women who slept seven hours a night. The less sleep women had, the more likely they were to gain weight. A lack of sleep increases levels of cortisol (a stress hormone), lowers leptin (leading to greater appetite), and increases ghrelin (which further stimulates appetite).

Many people compensate for poor sleep by eating a lot of sugary foods and drinking caffeinated beverages, which further disrupt normal sleep patterns. Large amounts of caffeine in particular mimic symptoms of anxiety and, when combined with stress, make a good night's rest all the more difficult. Although prescription medications can help to induce sleep, they come with side effects (such as middle-of-the-night refrigerator raids and "sleep-driving") and do not correct the real causes of sleep disorders.

Loud snoring and sleep apnea are almost always related to prediabetes or excess weight. Food allergies may also be a factor—foods you crave or consume in the evening should be considered possible food allergens. Losing weight and improving your blood-sugar levels will almost always help both your snoring and your sleep apnea.

Avoid overeating at dinnertime. Instead, aim to feel pleasantly full but not stuffed, and avoid snacking after dinner. Allergies or not, late-night snacking will affect your blood-sugar levels in the morning. It's better to wake up hungry and eat breakfast than to wake up without any interest in food and then skip breakfast.

Supplements That Might Help You Sleep Better

The first step in resolving sleep disorders, snoring, and sleep apnea is to avoid junk foods, improve your blood-sugar levels, and lose weight. Eliminate or at least greatly reduce your consumption of caffeinated beverages. Avoid taking any supplements with vitamin B6 later than midafternoon because large amounts of this vitamin can stimulate vivid dreams.

These supplements might help you sleep better.

- *Melatonin*, 250 mcg to 9 mg daily. This hormone, which you can buy without a prescription at most health food stores and pharmacies, regulates your sleep cycle. The time that you take it, however, and the dosage are critical. If you take too much or take it at the wrong time of day, it will leave you feeling groggy. Start with about 250 mcg, about two hours before bedtime. If it doesn't make you drowsy, increase the dose to 500 mcg the next evening. The effective dose varies widely between individuals, and you can safely work your way up to 9 mg (9,000 mcg), if necessary. Do not drive after taking melatonin, and do not use any sharp objects or other tools that might cause injury. If you feel groggy the next day, you have taken too much.

- *Tryptophan* or *5-hydroxytryptophan (5-HTP)*. These are two slightly different forms of the principal building block of serotonin, a neurotransmitter that helps us to feel relaxed. Try taking 50 to 100 mg of 5-HTP about one hour before bed. Alternatively, you can also take 500 to 2,000 mg of tryptophan before bed. Start with the lower dosage.

Getting a good night's sleep isn't just about foods and capsules, even natural ones. After about 8 p.m., start to reduce sensory stimulation in your environment by dimming the lights, listening to soft music, reading, and turning off the computer and the television (or at least lowering the volume). In other words, follow a transition from being awake to being asleep, instead of simply trying to go to sleep.

Mood Swings, Fuzzy Thinking, and Blood Sugar

Are you moody, or do you have trouble concentrating? The brain functions at its best when blood-sugar levels fall within a fairly narrow and relatively stable range. Rapid fluctuations in blood sugar can alter mood and behavior long before other health problems appear.

The moods of some people follow the ups and downs of their blood-sugar levels. Almost everyone feels pretty good, contented, and upbeat after eating—that is, when their blood sugar is up. Conversely, some people feel irritable, dissatisfied, or depressed when they delay or skip a meal—when their blood sugar is down. When blood-sugar levels are low, the activity of "higher" brain areas shuts down, and brain areas involved in more aggressive behavior become active. In ancient times, low blood sugar was a clear signal to hunt or gather food.

People who are prediabetic or overweight are more likely than thin people to feel anxious or depressed. There are likely a variety of reasons for this. The eating habits that shape overweight and prediabetes tend to be low in neuronutrients—that is, protein and B-complex vitamins, which are involved in making mood-regulating neurotransmitters. Meanwhile, overweight people may not like their appearance; they might feel anxious about how they look in public or feel depressed because they cannot change how they look.

In addition, people who are prediabetic, diabetic, or overweight are also more likely to have difficulty in concentrating and thinking clearly, especially after eating, when their blood sugar is elevated. Postmeal increases in blood sugar suppress brain levels of orexins, a family of brain chemicals that is responsible for making us feel alert. Abnormally high glucose levels (not low blood sugar) and low levels of orexins are why many people feel sleepy after eating. Long-term, having diabetes and being overweight increase the risk of developing Alzheimer's disease.

Supplements That Might Help with Moodiness

Emphasizing a diet of fish, lean protein, and high-fiber vegetables should improve your moods and mental clarity. If you have mood swings, be vigilant about avoiding sugary foods and any other kind of junk food.

- *B-complex vitamins*, in the form of a high-potency supplement, should help as well. For in-depth advice on improving your mood with supplements, foods, and lifestyle changes, see Jack's previous book *The Food-Mood Solution*. Carlson's Mellow Mood supplement contains B vitamins with GABA and "Suntheanine."
- *Chromium* has been found to relieve depression in people who also have eating disorders. Other supplements that enhance glucose control are likely to help as well. Try 500 mcg of chromium polynicotinate or chromium picolinate daily.

Supplements That Might Help with Fuzzy Thinking

Eating more protein and fewer sugars and carbs, particularly for breakfast and lunch, may help to keep your mind focused. In addition, try these supplements.

- *B-complex vitamins*, in the form of a high-potency supplement.
- *Omega-3 fish oils*, 2 to 3 grams daily.
- *GABA*, 200 mg daily. Gamma amino butyric acid, an amino acid and neurotransmitter, helps your brain to filter out distractions.
- *L-theanine*, 100 mg twice daily. This amino acid, found in green tea, both relaxes you and improves your mental focus. Look for "Suntheanine" on the label as a sign of quality.
- *Pycnogenol*, an antioxidant, 100 mg daily. This supplement has been found helpful in treating hyperactive behavior.

Heartburn, Gastroesophageal Reflux Disease, and Obesity

Since the mid-1990s, pharmaceutical companies have transformed heartburn into gastroesophageal reflux disease (GERD). By some estimates, 20 percent of people in North America have GERD. Whether that number is accurate or inflated, one thing is certain: each year, people get billions of dollars' worth of prescriptions for Prilosec, Nexium, and related drugs.

Has there been a genuine increase in heartburn and GERD? We believe there has been, mainly because of a deterioration in healthy eating habits and an increase in the number of overweight people. One would think that both doctors and patients would recognize that heartburn and GERD, which are caused by poor eating habits, are best treated by improving one's eating habits.

Virtually everyone experiences heartburn at one time or another. GERD is typically diagnosed when heartburn occurs frequently. Technically, the condition develops when the lower esophageal sphincter, a valvelike muscle, becomes weak and cannot prevent stomach acid from regurgitating upward. People who are overweight have a higher risk of suffering from GERD, and that risk increases with the amount of weight. Modest increases in weight, even when within normal ranges, can make people more likely to develop GERD.

Episodes of heartburn and GERD are usually caused by people eating too much food, resulting in a backflow (or reflux) of stomach acid into the esophagus. In more blunt terms, the conditions result from pigging out. A large study at the University of Arizona medical school found that the consumption of soft drinks was strongly associated with nighttime heartburn. Food allergies or sensitivities likely play a role, along with inadequate levels of digestive enzymes. If you usually develop heartburn or GERD after eating particular foods, stop eating those foods!

Untreated, chronic heartburn and GERD can develop into Barrett's esophagus, a precancerous condition, and nighttime heartburn is particularly damaging to the esophagus. But conventional acid-suppressing drugs carry their own risks. Regularly using any type of acid-suppressing drug almost doubles your risk of contracting pneumonia. The reason may be related to a suppression of gut bacteria, which help to protect against infection. People who use Prilosec, Nexium, and other types of acid-reducing drugs are more likely to experience hip fractures. The risk is significant—almost a 50 percent increase of hip fracture after one year, and two and one-half times greater risk of fracture after long-term use of the drug.

Normally, the acid environment of the stomach helps to break food down for further digestion. Throughout the digestive tract, hundreds of species of good bacteria also help to break down food, enhance immune function, and protect us from infection. Acid-suppressing drugs alter the environment within the digestive tract. They increase our risk of developing atrophic gastritis, which throws a wrench into the absorption of vitamin B12, vitamin C, and likely many other nutrients. They may also reduce calcium absorption, which would explain the greater risk of having a hip fracture.

Recent studies have found that imbalances among different species of gut bacteria can increase the risk of obesity. The imbalances favor gut bacteria that help to break down otherwise indigestible food constituents, leading to the absorption of more calories. It is very possible that oral antibiotics, which disrupt gut bacteria, also promote obesity.

Supplements That Might Help to Reduce Your Risk of Heartburn and GERD

Heartburn and GERD are actually signs of an abused digestive tract. The first step in correcting the problem is to follow our dietary recommendations and emphasize fresh, wholesome foods. At the same time, avoid processed foods containing sugar, refined carbohydrates, and trans fats.

Several types of supplements, available at health food stores, can help to heal the gut. These supplements include the following.

- *Probiotics*, which are supplements that contain beneficial bacteria. Follow the label directions for use.
- *Digestive enzymes*, which supplement those that your body makes. Follow the label directions for use. If you have an ulcer, however, do not take digestive aids until your ulcer heals.
- *Swedish bitters* and *artichoke leaf extract* are helpful for occasional heartburn or stomach upset. Follow the label directions for use.

The next chapter focuses on how moderately increased physical activity can help you to lower your blood-sugar and insulin levels, as well as reduce your weight.

12

Get More Active and Actually Enjoy It

E veryone knows that exercise is good for one's health, and everyone also understands the problem with it. Most people hate to exercise; they even hate the thought of it. Only a minority of people engages in any kind of regular exercise. The rest are die-hard couch potatoes who don't have the motivation to walk farther than to their refrigerator.

The situation has gotten even worse in recent years, with jobs in developed countries becoming more sedentary than ever. The average American now watches four and one-half hours of television each day. When you add the time people spend e-mailing, surfing the Internet, and listening to the radio, it amounts to almost ten hours a day of sitting around. Fingers might get a great workout on keyboards and remote controls, but the rest of the body doesn't.

Because so many people have a negative attitude toward the very word *exercise*, we almost always recommend increased *physical activity*. We hope this chapter motivates you to get moving with either a regular habit of physical activity or a more structured exercise program. Combined with better eating habits and taking supplements, greater physical activity will give you the upper hand in controlling your blood sugar, insulin, and weight.

Are we trying to trick you into exercising by using a more palatable term? The difference between exercise and physical activity is more than simple semantics. For many people, exercise conjures up all sorts of unpleasant images, such as feeling sweaty, wiped out, and embarrassed in front of other people.

If you have not been exercising, physical activity has many advantages over exercise. It allows you to start at an easy and comfortable pace. Physical activity doesn't have to be as structured as exercise, although it can and should be something you engage in most days of the week. Nor does physical activity require much in the way of preparation, time, money, or equipment. Physical activity accommodates your style and your routine, not that of a trainer, a gym, or a competitive athlete.

That's not to say we have anything against more rigorous exercise. To the contrary, the more activity you engage in (within reason), the better off you'll be in the long run. But we realize that asking you to do too much too soon would be a turnoff, and that's the last thing we want to do. Think of physical activity as a series of small steps. You'll take bigger steps when you're ready.

The Benefits of Physical Activity

The health benefits of physical activity are in many ways comparable to those of better eating habits. Moderate physical activity complements good eating habits and is much safer than any medication.

- *Physical activity lowers blood-sugar levels.* There's no question that greater physical activity improves blood-sugar levels, and the types of activities do not have to be strenuous. Many studies have shown that just going for a daily walk can lower blood-sugar, cholesterol, and triglyceride levels. One study found impressive benefits in both blood sugar and insulin after a single seventy-five-minute walk.

- *Physical activity lowers insulin levels.* Increased physical activity also improves the ability of insulin to do its job. As a result, your body needs to make less insulin, which lowers your risk of developing diabetes, heart disease, cancer, and many other diseases. Again, just going for a daily walk can reduce your insulin levels.

- *Physical activity shrinks the size of fat cells.* Once fat cells accumulate around your belly, it's difficult to permanently get rid of them. You can shrink the size of those fat cells, though, which is almost as good. Combining physical activity with a diet of protein and vegetables (and relatively few sugars and starches) helps to burn fat and shrink fat cells.

- *Physical activity reduces the risk of developing diabetes and other diseases.* Moderate levels of physical activity lower your risk of developing diabetes, regardless of how much you weigh. The benefits of activity protect you against other diseases as well. In the last few years, two dozen studies have found that moderate physical activity lowers the risk of heart disease by 18 to 84 percent, stroke by 21 to 34 percent, cancer by 30 to 40 percent, and dementia by 15 to 50 percent. Because of the reduction of disease risk, people live longer. In people over age fifty, moderate-to-high levels of physical activity increase life expectancy from about one and one-half to three and one-half years for both men and women.

Two More Reasons to Increase Your Physical Activity

As people get older, their muscle mass decreases and this eventually results in physical frailty and a higher risk of falling and fractures. This age-related muscle loss further impairs glucose tolerance, making you even more susceptible to prediabetes and diabetes. The consequences are much worse if you are already prediabetic or diabetic. This inevitable decrease in muscle mass can be slowed in several ways, however, such as by eating adequate amounts of protein, engaging in regular physical activity, and taking supplements of vitamin D and leucine (which we also discuss in this chapter).

In addition, following a low-calorie diet without at least moderate levels of physical activity will lead to the loss of both muscle and bone. That's because weight loss results from a decrease of both fat and muscle. As we explained in our discussion of protein in chapter 4, however, protein-rich eating habits do a better job of preserving muscle mass in comparison with simple low-calorie diets.

Protein-rich diets can also help to preserve bone mass and bone density, as long as the diet includes large amounts of vegetables and fruits.

Protein is necessary for the formation of both muscle and bone, and eating vegetables and fruit counteracts any potential negative impact from consuming large amounts of protein.

SALLY'S STORY
Correcting Midlife Hormone Imbalances

Sometimes a perimenopausal woman will show signs of three interrelated hormone problems: high insulin, low estrogen, and low thyroid. That was the case with Sally, who had been petite most of her life but had gained thirty pounds in her midfifties. She was embarrassed by all the extra weight around her tummy and rear end, even though she was an avid bicyclist.

The weight gain that is often characteristic of menopause may be related to low thyroid as well as to low estrogen. Both hormones tend to decline in women in their early to midfifties. Although research is limited, high levels of insulin are sometimes associated with low thyroid hormone activity, with the combination also encouraging weight gain.

Lab tests confirmed that Sally's estrogen levels and thyroid activity were low. She also had moderately elevated fasting blood sugar (95) and fasting insulin (14 mcIU/ml) levels, suggestive of prediabetes. Although the exercise probably helped to control her blood sugar, all of the energy bars and drinks she consumed most likely boosted her insulin levels.

Treatment included a bioidentical estrogen product and Armour's natural-source thyroid hormone (which contains both of the major thyroid hormones). Meanwhile, Sally's supplement plan included a high-potency multivitamin, a multimineral, and extra iodine and selenium, which are needed for normal thyroid function. She improved her eating habits, relying more on fruit and water instead of energy bars and drinks while cycling. After six months, she had lost fifteen pounds and gained more energy, finishing her first "century" (hundred-mile) bike ride.

Nutrition and Physical Activity: Is One Better Than the Other?

Nutrition is better than physical activity when it comes to losing significant amounts of weight. The reason is that it takes a lot of time and effort to burn calories, and it takes even longer if you have had a habit of eating a large number of calories. For example, to burn off the 670 calories in a Burger King Original Whopper, you would have to walk for almost three hours, cycle for more than one and one-half hours, or jog for a little more than one hour. Similarly, it would take almost an hour of walking to burn off the 210 calories in a Subway turkey breast sandwich. Most people don't have that much time after each meal, so it's far more effective to combine a lower intake of carbohydrate calories with more physical activity.

Physical activity is better than nutrition when it comes to increasing muscle, firming up sagging skin, and sculpting your body. Protein provides the nutrients needed to make muscle, but activity stimulates the conversion of dietary protein to muscle protein. When you're physically active, muscle cells become more active metabolically, enabling them to burn more blood sugar and fat. That's important because muscle cells burn most of the carbs and the fat that you consume. With regular physical activity, you increase the amount of muscle in your body, which means you end up with more glucose- and fat-burning cells.

QUICK TIP

Two Ways to Stick with Your Program

About nine out of ten people who increase their physical activity stop after about a month and a half. The most common reasons are injuries and a lack of social reinforcement. To combat the first problem, start with a low-risk activity, such as walking—and be careful where you step. Your stamina will noticeably improve after a couple of weeks or so. For the second problem, invite a family member, a friend, or a coworker to join you. Or get an energetic dog that needs to be walked every day.

When combined with improved eating habits, greater physical activity has an "additive" benefit that promotes weight loss. Donald K. Layman, Ph.D., of the University of Illinois, Urbana, and his colleagues placed forty-eight overweight middle-age women on one of two diets—one high protein and low carbohydrate, and the other low protein and high carbohydrate. Some of the women from each group also participated in regular exercise. Although all of the women lost weight, those on the high-protein diet plus exercise lost the most body fat while maintaining the most lean muscle mass. They lost more than 20 percent of their body fat in four months. In contrast, those on the high-carbohydrate diet who didn't exercise lost only 12.8 percent of their body fat.

Overcoming the Top Five Excuses

People come up with a lot of reasons for not being more physically active, and odds are that you have, too. It might surprise you, but nearly everyone's excuses boil down to the same five. Here are the most common excuses, along with our thoughts.

1. *I'm too tired.* Being tired all the time is often a sign of prediabetes. Do nothing and we'll guarantee that your energy levels will get even worse. That said, you might feel a little more tired immediately after physical activity during the first few days or couple of weeks of making a concerted effort to be more active. Feeling tired after physical activity means that you've pushed yourself a little, and that's good. It

---

QUICK TIP

Don't Make Exercise a Stress-Filled Activity

Some people stress themselves out by how they exercise. They might get up too early, push themselves too hard, or be anxious about leaving work and getting to the gym by a certain time. Even though physical activity requires exertion, it can be a time to mentally relax or think. You can go for a walk and talk with your spouse, or go for a slow and easy bicycle ride.

also means that you have begun a transition from getting sicker to getting healthier.

During this time, it's important to stay well within your comfort zone and not push yourself too hard. Start with a short walk, maybe ten or fifteen minutes. Your blood sugar and insulin will start to improve right away, and your stamina will increase within a couple of weeks. It just takes a little longer for your muscles to acclimate and strengthen, but you'll notice an improvement pretty fast.

2. *I don't have enough time.* Nearly everyone feels overwhelmed by everything they have to do at home or work, and people often feel as if they can't add another thing to their busy lives. As with everything else, making the time (or not) for physical activity is a choice. You probably have time to talk on the phone and watch your favorite television shows, so why not for a little more physical activity?

Engaging in some sort of physical activity, even for a few minutes, can actually clear your head, enabling you to refocus and prioritize all the other things you have to do. Fitting a new commitment into your busy schedule is a matter of being mindful of your need to be active, just as you are mindful of what you eat. Short bursts of activity are as effective as long stretches of activity. So if you're driving to the mall, park in a more distant spot. If you work in an office building, take a little break and walk up and down a couple of flights of stairs.

3. *I'd be embarrassed.* You might feel embarrassed by being overweight or out of shape. If you don't do anything, you'll still be overweight and out of shape. Worse, being diagnosed as prediabetic or diabetic is pretty embarrassing—it's like wearing a sign that says you failed to take care of yourself.

When you become more physically active, most other people will recognize that you're working at getting back into shape. If you're very shy or really concerned about your appearance, you can use small hand weights, a stationary bicycle, or a treadmill in the privacy of your home, or walk in your neighborhood or at a shopping mall. You never have to exercise while wearing skimpy clothing.

4. *I don't know how to begin.* At some point you didn't know how to drive a car or use a computer, yet you learned. Being more physically

active is like acquiring any new skill. Your balance, agility, and strength quickly start to improve—and so will your self-esteem. Again, early on, don't overdo.

5. *I get bored exercising.* Any type of physical activity can be boring if you approach it as a chore and do it by yourself. Find an activity that you'll enjoy. One way to overcome boredom is to exercise with another person, so that you can talk while walking or cycling. If you live alone, use a stationary bicycle or other exercise equipment while watching television. If you're out walking, you can listen to podcasts or music on your MP3 player—just pay attention to your surroundings, the traffic, and any hazards you might trip over. You can also vary your activities, walking one day, sweeping the garage or the driveway on another, and working with hand weights the next.

The Different Types of Physical Activity

Physical activities and exercise are often grouped by what they do for the body. It's good to know the different types. The two principal types of activities are aerobics and strength-training (resistance) exercises. There's always a little overlap between the two kinds.

Aerobic activities oxygenate the body's tissues, particularly the muscles, the heart, and the lungs, which in turn promotes the burning of glucose and fat. Aerobic activities can include brisk walking, high-intensity dancing (such as Jazzercize), rowing, and high-speed cycling. These activities help to reduce the risk of developing diabetes and heart disease.

Strength training forces the muscles to work against the resistance of another object. Weight lifting and body building are forms of resistance exercises. So is rowing, which builds both arm and leg muscles. Resistance exercises can sculpt your body by firming up the muscles in your torso, arms, and legs.

Researchers have found that regular short bursts of activity (such as sprinting, dancing, or chopping wood) are every bit as good as endurance exercises (such as jogging or long-distance cycling).

Why We Recommend Walking

Because you are likely prediabetic or overweight, we recommend that you start with safe, low-intensity physical activities. These include walking, easy-paced cycling, swimming, and working with hand weights. You can supplement these activities with occasional sweeping, vacuuming, and walking up and down stairs.

Walking is by far our top choice for people who have been sedentary. You can walk practically anywhere, such as in your neighborhood, at a shopping mall, or in a park. You can do it practically any time: in the early morning, during your lunch break, or after dinner. It doesn't cost anything because you don't need specialized equipment, although a good pair of shoes will make it easy on your feet. You can control and change your level of effort by walking faster or slower or by walking on a level surface or uphill.

It may surprise you, but walking downhill (and, similarly, walking down a flight of stairs) does a better job of improving glucose tolerance than walking uphill does. A study by Heinz Drexel, M.D., of the Academic Hospital in Feldkirch, Austria, compared the effects of walking uphill or downhill. The subjects in his study, all healthy, walked either up- or downhill, with about a two-thousand-foot change in elevation, three to five times a week for two months. Walking uphill, which most people feel is more strenuous, resulted in a 9 percent improvement in glucose tolerance. Walking downhill, however, improved glucose tolerance by 25 percent.

Drexel's finding seems counterintuitive. Why would an easier walk improve glucose tolerance more than a strenuous one does? The reason is that walking uphill shortens muscle cells; the shortening occurs in response to lifting a weight, such as your body or barbells. In contrast, when muscle cells resist a force, such as gravity, they stretch out. It is possible that longer muscle cells use more glucose compared with shorter muscle cells.

Wear a pair of shoes that offer both comfort and a good grip. They might be advertised as walking, jogging, tennis, or cross-trainer shoes. They should fit comfortably, and you should also wear thicker socks instead of thin ones. A rubberlike sole will grip sidewalks and

Physical Activity and the Time of Day

Many people exercise in the early morning before going to work; how-ever, engaging in physical activity between 2 p.m. and 4 p.m. has an advantage. Body temperature at this time of day is about two degrees higher than in the morning, and that means you'll feel warmer and your muscles will be more flexible. Your reaction times will be faster, you'll feel stronger, and activity will require less exertion, compared with in the morning. Test whether evening exercise works for you. It relaxes some people but stimulates others.

the occasionally slippery mall surface. Leather-soled shoes may slip on some surfaces.

Note: If you are diabetic, check the bottoms of your feet daily for any sign of injury. People with diabetes have a higher risk of developing foot numbness (diabetic neuropathy), which may prevent them from feeling foot injuries.

Consider buying a digital pedometer, which may cost $5 to $30, depending on its features (most of which you won't need). Pedometers clip to your belt, and they record the number of steps you take. Aim for 2,000 to 3,000 steps, and work your way up to 5,000 and then 10,000 steps daily.

Increase your speed and distance as you feel comfortable, but do not run. You may initially feel a little out of breath. It's all right to stop and rest. You're not in a race.

Always walk where you feel safe. This could be near your home, where you work, or in a mall. Always pay attention to traffic and any person who might be following you.

Measuring Your Benefits

Your doctor can periodically measure your fasting blood-sugar and insulin levels to track your progress. As a general rule, any decrease in blood-sugar and insulin levels is good and, over the long run, will lower your risk of developing complications and other diseases.

There are a couple of ways to track your own progress without medical tests. First, pay attention to how long you walked (swam, cycled, etc.) before feeling tired. You should be able to increase your distance or speed a little each week.

Second, if you are overweight, you will most likely lose weight while following our dietary and activity recommendations. At some point, however, your weight loss may plateau or even increase a little. This is often perplexing or frustrating to dieters, but it might actually reflect some positive changes.

Here's why. Muscle weighs more than fat, so if you increase the amount of muscle you have, your weight may remain the same or increase slightly. For this reason, we recommend that you forego the scale and periodically check your waist size with a cloth tape measure. Your waist size may go down, along with your body proportions, such as your waist-hip ratio, regardless of your weight.

Can Any Supplements Help with Exercise?

A few nutritional supplements might actually improve how efficiently your body makes muscle, as well as increase your energy levels. These supplements may enhance your ability to be physically active, but they are not substitutes for activity.

- *Vitamin D.* We have already recommended that you take a daily capsule containing at least 1,000 IU of vitamin D. This vitamin is essential for normal glucose tolerance, but it's nearly impossible to get adequate amounts from foods. Your body needs vitamin D to make muscles. It won't turn you into Superman, but combined with physical activity it will help your body to make normal amounts of muscle.

- *Leucine.* This protein building block is found in fish, meat, and chicken. Like vitamin D, it seems to enhance the body's production of muscle but via a different mechanism. Although you will get plenty of leucine by following our dietary recommendations, you might consider trying supplemental branched-chain amino acids, which would include leucine, isoleucine, and valine. Follow the label directions for use.

- *B vitamins.* If you take a high-potency multivitamin or Carlson's Nutra-Support Diabetes supplement, you'll get the B-complex vitamins. They play numerous roles in energy-producing reactions.
- *CoQ10.* This vitaminlike nutrient plays crucial roles in helping the body use food for energy. Take 30 to 100 mg.
- *Carnitine.* This vitaminlike nutrient is found in animal protein, and it helps cells to burn fat for energy. Take 500 to 1,000 mg.

By increasing your physical activity in small but consistent ways, you will help your body do a better job of lowering blood sugar, cholesterol, and triglycerides. As your muscle increases, and your carbohydrate calories decrease, your body will also start to burn belly fat. You will feel better physically, and you will gain a newfound sense of accomplishment.

13

The Four-Week Stop Prediabetes Now Plan

Whenwe talk with individuals or lecture groups about prediabetes, we find that most people are very motivated to regain and maintain their health. They have had a taste of poor health, and they don't like it! Almost always, one of their first questions is about how to actually begin improving their eating habits and lifestyle. Another common question is about how to stick with a dietary plan.

In this final chapter we outline our four-week Stop Prediabetes Now plan. Its purpose is simple: to help you organize and put into practice what you have learned about improving your eating habits, reversing prediabetes, and controlling your weight. You don't have to follow the steps in the order described here, but doing so may provide a helpful structure and may enable you to achieve faster and better benefits.

The key steps are spread over four weeks so you don't feel overwhelmed by the many changes in your eating habits. Each week includes important steps for you to take, along with ways to track your progress. You can also speed up or slow down the plan, making the dietary and lifestyle changes in two weeks or in eight weeks.

You may want to photocopy some of the following pages, so that you have a ready reminder at home and at work and can make notes. It will also help you to occasionally refer back to earlier chapters, including those on reading labels, shopping at the supermarket, and ordering in restaurants.

You will sometimes ask yourself, "What can I eat?" For this reason, each of the four weeks includes daily meal plans. These meal plans are not meant to be a list or a sequence that you must rigidly follow. Rather, they are suggestions for healthy breakfasts, lunches, and dinners—an idea generator, so to speak. Use them as a menu of options for cooking at home or for eating out. If you prefer to eat chicken instead of fish, you can certainly eat more chicken and less fish. It is important, however, regardless of what you eat, to follow the dietary principles and guidelines in chapter 5.

How do you stay motivated? We believe there are several factors that influence motivation. One is the enjoyment of life that comes with feeling better, physically and mentally, after you adopt healthier eating habits. Gaining better mental focus and having more energy will likely be among the first improvements you'll notice. In fact, you may feel better than you have in years. Recovering your health is a powerful motivator for staying healthy.

To keep on track, be mindful of what you eat and develop a personal discipline or a routine that governs what you choose to eat and not to eat. Being mindful means to be "in the moment" and also to be aware of potential consequences of your actions. It's certainly easy to eat a fast-food meal or a pizza, whereas it takes (at least early on) a conscious effort to opt for healthier foods. After a few weeks or a couple of months, however, your new style of eating will feel like second nature.

You can, of course, make a habit of cheating on your diet and admonishing yourself. Many people do, and we won't be looking over your shoulder saying, "You shouldn't eat that." But if you cheat on a regular basis, you are only cheating yourself of good health. Your prediabetes will lead to diabetes, and diabetes is a terrible disease—in its later stages, as terrible as cancer or congestive heart failure. Habitual cheating also points to powerful food addictions. If you have a history of being a diet cheater, you may want to revisit the section on food addictions in chapter 3.

What should you do if you occasionally fall "off the wagon" and eat unhealthy foods, such as a rich dessert? It is essential that later the same day or the next, you resume your healthier eating habits and emphasize lean protein. The protein will stabilize your blood sugar and, in doing so, will reduce your cravings for unhealthy foods.

Before You Begin

To track your progress, you need a starting reference point. So before you begin our program, ask your physician to conduct several blood tests, which are objective measures of your health. It's very possible that you recently had these tests:

- Fasting glucose
- Fasting insulin
- Triglycerides
- High-sensitivity C-reactive protein
- HbA_{1c}

Get a copy of your test results from your doctor's office and keep them in a safe place. Compare your results with the ranges we describe in chapter 1, and gauge your progress in future tests as well.

You can also benefit from several subjective measurements at home. You'll need a scale and a cloth tape measure, as we described in chapter 1. These measurements include

- Your body weight
- Your body mass index
- Your waist-hip ratio

Many of your other subjective benchmarks will be related to how you feel, such as your energy levels and ability to concentrate. Consider keeping a brief daily diary with notes of what you eat and how you feel before and after each meal.

Week 1

This is a transitional week, reflecting the beginning of your shift from disease-promoting to health-promoting eating habits. Odds are that you have already begun to improve your eating habits. We recommend that you tackle what needs to be done on a day when you have plenty of time to spend shopping and in your kitchen. With the knowledge you have gained from earlier chapters, here's what we would like you to do.

- *Clean out your pantry, refrigerator, and freezer.* Throw out any foods and beverages that contain sugar, including sucrose, fructose, corn syrup, and high-fructose corn syrup. Next, throw out all foods that are made with partially or fully hydrogenated oils. Look specifically for the word *hydrogenated* on labels because the types of oil may differ. In addition, dispose of all foods that contain shortening, corn oil, soybean oil, wheat, or flour.

  You may be shocked by how much food you'll throw out. Reversing prediabetes means that you must emphasize fresh over packaged foods. If you hate the thought of wasting all this food, try to return whatever you can to the store where you bought it. You can also donate nonperishable foods to many charitable organizations and churches, but we have ethical reservations about giving unhealthy foods to poor people. However you choose to dispose of these foods, get them out of the house, and make no excuses for keeping or eating them.

- *Do some meal planning.* Many people don't think about their next meal until they are hungry. That's the worst time to go shopping or eat in a restaurant. When you're hungry, it's all too easy to eat unhealthy foods that promote prediabetes and weight gain.

  Give some thought to what you would like to prepare and eat over the next two to three days. You might start by looking for several recipes that appeal to you, or maybe you've already got a favorite recipe that you can modify with healthier ingredients. Think in terms of high-quality protein (such as fish, chicken, or lean meat) and fresh vegetables. Unless you engage in strenuous exercise, skip all carbs (except those naturally found in vegetables) during the first week.

- *Create a shopping list.* Divide your shopping list into three parts: staples, "back-up foods," and ingredients for meals. Taking this approach will streamline your future shopping trips.

For staples, include whatever ingredients you'll regularly use, such as olive oil, dried herbs and spices, and eggs. Refer to our list of kitchen staples in chapter 8. We also like to have some back-up foods, such as cheese and deli turkey (or leftovers), for when we're pressed for time and need a quick bite to eat. The last part of the shopping list should be ingredients for meals over the next two or three days.

Because week 1 is transitional, try to keep things simple, particularly if you haven't made a habit of cooking. Pan-fried fish or chicken breasts, homemade burgers, steamed vegetables, chicken salad, and salads are fine. Although fresh foods are best, it is all right to keep some frozen fish, chicken, and veggies in the freezer.

• *Use your first Sunday as a food-preparation and cooking day.* Food prep and cooking can and should be enjoyable and relaxing activities, so don't rush things. If you start in the morning, dice some veggies (such as red bell peppers and scallions) to include with scrambled eggs. Place extras in plastic storage containers, and use the diced peppers and scallions as toppings on salads.

For breakfast, consider making the Scrambled Egg and Vegetable Sauté (see the recipe on page 154), which allows for leftovers that can be reheated in a microwave oven on Monday and Tuesday morning. Later that day, you can roast a chicken or pan-fry a fish fillet or a chicken breast. Because food prep and cooking take time, get into the habit of making more than you'll eat in a single meal. Use the leftovers for subsequent meals, and you'll cook fewer days during the week.

Five Key Points to Remember while Following the Plan

1. Build most meals around a centerpiece of high-quality protein.

2. Eat protein with breakfast every day.

3. Include some high-fiber vegetables or fruit with each meal.

4. Include some vinegar, grapefruit, and cinnamon each day.

5. Eat smaller portions for lunch and dinner than you have in the past.

Sample Meal Plan for Week 1

An asterisk (*) means the recipe is in this book. You can find many other recipes in Jack's other books (including *Feed Your Genes Right* and *The Inflammation Syndrome*), in cookbooks, and on the Internet. To get you into the habit of eating a protein-rich breakfast, we recommend that you prepare the first breakfast on a Sunday morning, refrigerating and reheating the leftovers for breakfast on Monday and Tuesday. As a general rule, try to cook enough food so that you have leftovers that can be easily reheated—this will save time and effort with at least one subsequent meal.

Sunday (Day 1)

Breakfast	Scrambled Egg and Vegetable Sauté* and fresh fruit
Lunch	Curried Chicken Salad* on a bed of chopped lettuce
Dinner	Pan-Fried Salmon* with bok choy sautéed in olive oil and tamari (wheat-free soy sauce)

Monday (Day 2)

Breakfast	Reheated Scrambled Egg and Vegetable Sauté*
Lunch	Chicken Caesar salad (without croutons)
Dinner	Sautéed Scallops with Saffron Sauce* and sautéed snow peas

Tuesday (Day 3)

Breakfast	Reheated Scrambled Egg and Vegetable Sauté*
Lunch	Soup and salad
Dinner	Mediterranean-Style Pan-Fried Chicken Breasts* and vegetables

Wednesday (Day 4)

Breakfast	Omelet with diced ham, bell peppers, and cheese
Lunch	Chicken Caesar salad (without croutons)
Dinner	Sautéed Shrimp* and vegetables

Thursday (Day 5)

Breakfast	Scrambled eggs with diced chicken and cheese
Lunch	Roast beef and cheese slices and one apple
Dinner	Pan-Fried Tilapia (use recipe for Pan-Fried Salmon) with Pesto Sauce* and side salad

Friday (Day 6)

Breakfast	Italian-Style Omelet* with a side of berries
Lunch	Lamb Burger with Feta Cheese* and side salad
Dinner	Parmesan-encrusted halibut on a bed of arugula

Saturday (Day 7)

Breakfast	Ratatouille Omelet* with a side of apple slices
Lunch	Greek Salad*
Dinner	Shrimp Chipotle Fajitas*

Improvements You May Notice during Week 1

If you start to follow our dietary recommendations, you will likely feel better within a day or two. Although feeling better is a subjective measurement, it will reflect improvements in your blood sugar.

- Overall, you'll have more energy and feel sharper mentally.
- If you eat high-quality protein and veggies for lunch, you'll be less likely to feel tired in the early afternoon.
- By the end of the week, you'll notice that you have more energy and less mental fuzziness.
- It's possible that you'll lose a pound or two of weight by the end of week 1, but we don't recommend getting on a scale or taking out the tape measure just yet. You may notice, however, that your pants or skirts are a little bit looser.
- If you feel worse during the first few days, you may be withdrawing from food allergies or addictions, such as to foods made with wheat or dairy. If this is the case, your symptoms and cravings should ease after about five days. Refer back to the section on food allergies and addictions in chapter 3.

Week 2

Continue the eating habits you established in week 1. Meanwhile, review chapters 4 and 5, and incorporate some additional dietary recommendations. For example, if you still consume diet soft drinks, this would be a good time to switch to water and teas. Green tea, hot or iced, is particularly good because it slows the absorption of carbohydrates.

Add Nutritional Supplements to Your Plan

Week 2 is a good time to begin taking nutritional supplements (if you have not already done so) to enhance the beneficial effects of your new eating habits on your blood-sugar and insulin levels.

Start with a daily high-potency multivitamin-multimineral supplement. Some formulas will require that you take two or three capsules daily, and soft-gelatin capsules are easier than tablets to swallow. We recommend supplements from health or natural food stores because they typically have few troublesome additives, sweeteners, or colors. Make sure the supplement does not contain iron, unless your doctor has diagnosed you as iron deficient. A good option is Carlson's Nutra-Support Diabetes (visit www.carlsonlabs.com for more information). You can also purchase iron-free supplements from www.thorne.com.

Add at least one additional supplement that helps with blood-sugar or insulin levels. Consider taking (1) 100 mg of alpha-lipoic acid or R-lipoic acid fifteen minutes before each meal, or (2) 500 mcg of chromium polynicotinate with breakfast and dinner. In addition, take 100 to 200 mg of Pycnogenol daily.

Reduce Stress in Your Life

Stress increases the secretion of both insulin and the stress hormone cortisol, and together these hormones promote the formation of fat around the belly. Week 2 is a good time to tackle stress issues that affect your eating habits, moods, or sleep.

People's eating habits usually slide when they're stressed—they delay or skip meals, then succumb to fast foods. You can still manage a stressful job—and manage it better—by maintaining a semblance of good eating habits. Try to keep some cheese and an apple in your office refrigerator or in a cooler in your car. Taking a ten-minute break to eat gives you a little time to unwind and stabilize your blood sugar—and it's all the more important if you are prediabetic.

Stress also disrupts restful sleep, and inadequate sleep increases cortisol levels and your risk of developing belly fat. Often, because people feel tired, they consume too much caffeine in the form of coffee, energy drinks, and soft drinks. Unfortunately, all that caffeine exacerbates the stress, leaving people too edgy to fall asleep at bedtime. If you must have caffeine to get going in the morning, limit yourself to two cups. After that, stick with water, green tea, or herbal teas.

Feeling stressed is often a sign that you do not have adequate personal boundaries protecting you against the excessive demands of work or other people. To reduce stress, it's important to set priorities in work and social activities, avoid multitasking, and establish clear boundaries so that you have time for yourself. For more information on combating stress, refer to Jack's previous book *The Food-Mood Solution*.

Sample Meal Plan for Week 2

Sunday (Day 8)

Breakfast	Crustless mushroom and ham quiche
Lunch	Salmon Burgers,* with a side of steamed or marinated white asparagus
Dinner	Roast Chicken* and vegetables

Monday (Day 9)

Breakfast	Omelet with artichoke hearts and chicken pieces
Lunch	Tuna Salad in a Lettuce Wrap*
Dinner	Healthy Chicken Schnitzel* and steamed fresh green beans

Tuesday (Day 10)

Breakfast	Ground turkey patty with one scrambled egg
Lunch	Avocado slices and baby shrimp with salsa
Dinner	Poached Salmon* with Cream Sauce* and vegetables

Wednesday (Day 11)

Breakfast	Eggs Benedict (without the muffin)
Lunch	Greek-Style Gyro (no pita)* and side salad
Dinner	Baked Cornish hens and vegetables

Thursday (Day 12)

Breakfast	Omelet with marinated asparagus spear pieces
Lunch	Hamburger (no bun)* and steamed cauliflower
Dinner	Halibut with Caper Sauce* and vegetables or a salad

Friday (Day 13)

Breakfast	Scrambled Eggs and Romano Cheese* with a side of fresh fruit
Lunch	Cobb salad
Dinner	Grilled Shrimp* and vegetables

Saturday (Day 14)

Breakfast	Omelet with chicken pieces and avocado slices
Lunch	Tomato and mozzarella cheese slices, sprinkled with basil
Dinner	Chicken Piccata* and vegetables

Improvements You May Notice during Week 2

By the end of week 2, most people feel as if they have come through a hazy tunnel and now have considerably more energy and mental focus. As good as you may feel, however, remember that you are still very sensitive to sugary and carb-rich foods. Your energy levels and mental focus will likely plummet if you happen to eat these foods. If that happens, eat one or two high-protein meals to get back on track.

By this time, almost everyone notices a modest but clear reduction in weight or body measurements.

Week 3

By week 3, with improvements now obvious in your eating habits and stress levels, you should have the time and energy to incorporate light but regular physical activity into your plan.

If you have been a couch potato, begin with a leisurely ten- to fifteen-minute walk (or more, if you have the time) each day. If the weather is not conducive to walking, drive to a shopping mall and walk there—however, focus on walking to keep up your pace, not on window shopping.

If you tend to get bored while walking, find a walking partner to talk with. You can also listen to music, podcasts, or audiobooks on your MP3 player. Many public libraries allow people to download books. If you walk outdoors, however, be aware of your surroundings and personal safety.

The more physical activity you engage in, the greater the benefits in terms of your blood-sugar and insulin levels. So plan to increase your walking time and distance over the coming weeks. You can also engage in other types of physical activity, such as cycling, swimming, using hand weights, or a mix of several types of activities to prevent boredom. Try to avoid talking on your cell phone while walking, though, because the distraction will slow down your pace.

By week 3, you might be able to include *small* amounts of starchy foods, such as brown rice or part of a baked sweet potato with your meals. If you have a problem limiting yourself to small portions, however, it's best to hold off eating such foods for at least two more weeks.

Sample Meal Plan for Week 3

Sunday (Day 15)

Breakfast	Scrambled eggs with diced avocado and cheese
Lunch	Salmon Burger* with homemade tartar sauce
Dinner	London Broil (flank steak)* and sautéed spinach and mushrooms

Monday (Day 16)

Breakfast	Omelet with artichoke hearts and sausage pieces
Lunch	Traditional chicken and egg salad, on a bed of lettuce and tomato slices
Dinner	Seared sesame seed-encrusted Ahi tuna and sautéed bok choy

Tuesday (Day 17)

Breakfast	Huevos rancheros (without the tortilla)
Lunch	Wilted spinach salad with blue cheese and walnut pieces
Dinner	Pan-Fried Chicken Breasts* with fresh rosemary and garlic with a side of steamed cauliflower, broccoli, and carrots

Wednesday (Day 18)

Breakfast	Eggs Benedict (without the muffin)
Lunch	Tuna salad
Dinner	Baked Cornish hens, Pan-Fried Eggplant Slices,* and sugar-free yogurt

Thursday (Day 19)

Breakfast	Omelet with chives and organic cream cheese
Lunch	Bowl of gazpacho
Dinner	Trout almondine with a side of sautéed fennel, olives, and raisins

Friday (Day 20)

Breakfast	Eggs scrambled with diced green chili and Red Leicester cheese
Lunch	Tomato stuffed with tuna salad
Dinner	Chicken fajitas (no tortilla)

Saturday (Day 21)

Breakfast	Omelet with chicken pieces and avocado slices
Lunch	Turkey salad and a small tossed green salad
Dinner	Chicken Piccata* and vegetables

Improvements You May Notice during Week 3

By the end of week 3, if you have adhered to our dietary recommendations, your blood sugar and weight should have improved significantly, and you should be able to wear slightly smaller clothes.

Often people describe having side benefits by this time. These side benefits vary greatly among people but may include a reduction of aches and pains and other annoying symptoms that they had thought were too minor to mention to a doctor.

Week 4

By week 4, you will be reaping most of the benefits from changing your eating and lifestyle habits. Many of the changes you've made should start to feel a bit more like regular habits.

Work on incorporating all of the dietary changes we recommended in earlier chapters. In addition, this would be a good time to increase your intake of organically grown vegetables and fruits, as well as free-range or grass-fed chicken and beef.

Sample Meal Plan for Week 4

Sunday (Day 22)

Breakfast	Denver omelet
Lunch	Spinach salad with chicken and walnut pieces
Dinner	Lamb Burger with Feta Cheese* seasoned liberally with cinnamon, oregano, and garlic and sautéed squash and eggplant

Monday (Day 23)

Breakfast   Eggs Benedict (without the muffin)

Lunch   Portobello Personal Pizza* and side salad

Dinner   Sautéed shrimp with artichoke hearts in Dijon mustard sauce, lightly steamed cauliflower, and ½ cup baked spaghetti squash

Tuesday (Day 24)

Breakfast   Corned beef hash with poached eggs and fresh fruit

Lunch   Flakes of Poached Salmon* on red-leaf lettuce salad

Dinner   Braised beef brisket and sautéed snow peas

Wednesday (Day 25)

Breakfast   Scrambled eggs with baby shrimp and tomato sauce

Lunch   Shrimp and cucumber salad

Dinner   Beef tenderloin roasted with garlic and rosemary and sautéed spinach and mushrooms

Thursday (Day 26)

Breakfast   Omelet with sautéed baby asparagus spears

Lunch   Greek-Style Gyro*

Dinner   Oriental-style sautéed pork strips, with snow peas, bok choy, and other vegetables, seasoned with diced ginger, garlic, and tamari

Friday (Day 27)

Breakfast   Poached eggs on baked Portobello mushroom

Lunch   Ground turkey meatloaf and vegetables or a salad

Dinner   Salmon cubes, onion, tomato, and red bell pepper broiled on skewers

Saturday (Day 28)

Breakfast   Poached eggs over baked mashed sweet potato

Lunch	Cold deli plate with sliced turkey, lean roast beef, cheese, and side salad
Dinner	Chicken in lemon, garlic, and rosemary marinade and a small Greek salad

Improvements You May Notice during Week 4

By the end of week 4, you will most likely have lost five pounds of weight and probably a little more than that. You will also have lost one to two inches of belly fat. That's pretty impressive, considering that you didn't count calories, grams of carbs, or glycemic index rankings.

Your doctor may feel that it's a little too early to return for another round of blood tests, but tell him or her that you would like to check your progress. Follow-up tests may be especially important if you have been taking metformin (Glucophage) to lower your blood-sugar levels or any drug (such as statins) to lower blood fats. With reductions in blood sugar and blood fats, you may need less of these medications, or your doctor may be able to wean you from them.

The tests we recommend at this point include

- Fasting glucose
- Fasting insulin
- Triglycerides
- High-sensitivity C-reactive protein

We haven't included the HbA_{1c} test because it provides a composite of blood-sugar levels over the previous six to eight weeks. You can test for it by the end of your second month.

Looking Ahead: The End of Your Second Month

If you did not return for blood tests at the end week 4, this would be a good time to do so. You can test for

- Fasting glucose
- Fasting insulin
- Triglycerides

- High-sensitivity C-reactive protein
- HbA$_{1c}$

People do have a tendency to let their discipline slide, even for a day or two, or rebel against their improved eating habits. Because of this, it's worthwhile to periodically reread or skim parts of the book. Doing so will reinforce what you've learned.

In addition, you may find at some point that your weight reaches a plateau. If you have been consistently more physically active, this may reflect an increase in muscle mass, which weighs more than fat. We recommend that you use a tape measure to check the size of your belly and your waist-hip ratio.

Afterword

We all make choices as we go through life, but the act of making choices presumes that we know that more than one option exists: to go fast or slow, to be good or bad, or to eat healthy or unhealthy foods.

Unfortunately, when it comes to nutrition, many of us have been unaware of, have forgotten, or have been blinded to all of our options. As a result, people have often made the wrong choices, which led to their developing prediabetes, becoming overweight, and suffering from other health problems.

Why didn't we know better? And why haven't we made better choices?

There are many reasons, and you're not to blame for all of them.

One, schools rarely teach anything substantive about nutrition, and this is also true of medical schools. In fact, elementary school, high school, and college cafeterias serve some of the worst food in terms of nutritional value. If no one ever taught you that there's a big nutritional difference between a salad and a bag of greasy fries, it's hard to blame you for eating the fries.

Two, fast-food restaurants and the manufacturers of other junk foods spend billions of dollars each year trying to convince people that their foods are irresistible. Many of these foods are in fact addictive through a variety of biological mechanisms. If you travel in the United States, it often seems as if the only food options are McDonald's, Burger King, Taco Bell, and other fast-food restaurants. Their presence blinds people to other options. These purveyors of bad nutrition lobby Congress and federal agencies to serve their financial interests instead of the health and basic nutritional needs of consumers.

Three, people have a habit of taking the path of least resistance, which is often the path of greatest convenience. When we're stressed and short of time—or just plain lazy—it's easier to buy and eat processed, packaged, and less nutritious foods than it is to shop for or make a healthier meal. Related to this, we also tend to be creatures of habit. We prefer to stick with what we like to eat and we don't have much sense of adventure when it comes to trying new foods. We stay in our comfort zone partly because of the power of food addictions to our favorite foods and partly because peas and corn seem more familiar than broccoli and spinach.

Four, we're especially good at rationalizing our bad habits even when we do know better. We convince ourselves that a soft drink here or a candy bar there won't really hurt us. People are very good at denying the bad stuff in life, at least until there's no avoiding it.

Given the dwindling numbers of thin and healthy people, it's clear that all of these forces have contributed to making people sicker rather than healthier.

What can you do to change things?

It would be easy to blame only the fast-food restaurants and junk-food companies. After all, they certainly share a lot of the responsibility for making foods that promote prediabetes and overweight.

But blaming is not an effective way to change your behavior or eating habits. Blame focuses on what you can't have, change, or control. In *Stop Prediabetes Now*, we have detailed the specific changes that are needed to improve your health. Instead of blaming, refocus on what *you* can get, change, and control. The only person you can really change and control is you.

By reaching this point of the book, you have also come to a turning point in your life. You are now fully aware of how poor eating habits led to your health problems. More important, you now understand the steps you must take. Knowledge is power, and you can use this power to reverse prediabetes and increase your energy and zest for life.

Are you ready to let go of the old ways that made you sick? You can do it—one choice at a time.

Today is the first day of the rest of your life. Please choose to make it a healthy life.

RESOURCES
for Supplements, Foods, and Additional Information

Finding Professional Help

Working with a nutritionally oriented physician or psychiatrist can usually help you to identify and improve your mood and behavior problems. The following organizations provide referral services.

Referral Organizations for Finding Nutritionally Oriented Physicians

American Association of Naturopathic Physicians
www.naturopathic.org

American College for Advancement in Medicine
www.acam.org

International Society for Orthomolecular Medicine
www.orthomed.org or centre@orthomed.org

Nutritionally (Biochemically) Oriented Medical Center

The Center for the Improvement of Human Functioning International
3100 N. Hillside Avenue
Wichita, KS 67219
(316) 682-3100
www.brightspot.org

Newsletters, Books, and Web Sites

Many publications provide excellent information on diet and supplements, although you may sometimes have to navigate contradictory information or ignore information that's inconsistent with the Stop Prediabetes Now plan.

The Nutrition Reporter™. This monthly newsletter, produced by Jack Challem (the coauthor of this book), summarizes recent research on vitamins, minerals, and herbs. The annual subscription rate is $27 ($48 CND for Canada, $40 U.S. funds for all other countries). For a sample issue, send a business-size self-addressed envelope, with postage for two ounces, to The Nutrition Reporter, P. O. Box 30246, Tucson, AZ 85751. Sample issues are also available at www.nutritionreporter.com.

The Food-Mood Solution (John Wiley & Sons, 2007), by Jack Challem. Blood-sugar levels, nutrient deficiencies and imbalances, and poor eating habits affect moods, resulting in irritability, depression, anxiety, and fuzzy thinking. This book describes a dietary and lifestyle approach to improving moods.

Feed Your Genes Right (John Wiley & Sons, 2005), by Jack Challem. This book focuses on how our genes depend on vitamins and other nutrients, and how we can make the most of our genetic inheritance and reduce the risk of disease.

The Inflammation Syndrome: The Complete Nutritional Program to Prevent and Reverse Heart Disease, Arthritis, Diabetes, Allergies, and Asthma (John Wiley & Sons, 2003, $14.95), by Jack Challem. With a diet plan similar to the one in *Stop Prediabetes Now*, this book is tailored to people with chronic inflammatory diseases.

Syndrome X: The Complete Nutritional Program to Prevent and Reverse Insulin Resistance (John Wiley & Sons, 2000, $14.95), by Jack Challem, Burton Berkson, M.D., Ph.D., and Melissa Diane Smith. This was the first consumer book on Syndrome X, and a national bestseller, covering one common form of prediabetes.

The Official *Stop Prediabetes Now* Web Site
www.stopprediabetesnow.com

The Official *Food-Mood Solution* Web Site
www.foodmoodsolution.com

Medline/PubMed
The world's largest searchable database of medical journal articles, providing free abstracts (summaries) of more than 8 million articles.
www.pubmed.gov

Merck Manual
The online edition of your physician's standard medical reference book.
www.merck.com

Nutrient Data Laboratory Food Composition
Type in nearly any food or food product, and you instantly get its nutritional breakdown per cup or 100 grams.
www.nal.usda.gov/fnic/foodcomp

USDA Data on Nutritional Deficiencies
You can quickly look up the percentage of people nationally or in individual states who consume the basic recommended amounts of individual nutrients and, conversely, the appalling numbers of Americans who do not. This is the source of the data for the graph on page 208.
www.ba.ars.usda.gov/cnrg/services/cnmapfr.html

Sources for Quality Nutritional Supplements

Thousands of companies sell proprietary brands of vitamins, minerals, and other types of nutritional supplements. We've found the following companies to have high-quality and reliable products.

Advanced Physicians Products

Founded by a nutritionally oriented physician, APP offers an extensive line of high-quality vitamin and mineral supplements. For more information, call (800) 220-7687 or go to www.nutritiononline.com.

Carlson Laboratories

Carlson Laboratories makes Nutra-Support Diabetes, a high-potency multi-vitamin-multimineral supplement formulated specifically for the nutritional needs of people with prediabetes and diabetes. The company also sells exceptional fish oil supplements, including a lemon-flavored cod liver oil, the widest selection of natural vitamin E products, and a broad range of other vitamin and mineral supplements. For more information, call (800) 323-4141 or go to www.carlsonlabs.com.

Insulow

This company sells Insulow, a unique product that combines the more biologically active "R" form of alpha-lipoic acid (an antioxidant) with biotin (a B vitamin). This combination of ingredients helps to regulate blood-sugar and insulin levels, which is particularly important for people with glucose-tolerance problems, prediabetes, and diabetes. For more information, call (407) 384-3388 or go to www.insulow.com.

InterHealth Nutraceuticals

InterHealth manufactures Chromate chromium polynicotinate, a popular form of chromium, which is sold by more familiar brand names. The company also makes and markets Super CitriMax, which combines chromium polynicotinate with calcium and potassium hydroxycitrates. Super CitriMax may reduce both appetite and weight by improving insulin function and glucose levels. For more information, call (800) 783-4636 or go to www.interhealthusa.com and www.supercitrimax.com.

Nutricology/Allergy Research Group

Nutricology/Allergy Research Group is often at the cutting edge of original nutritional supplement formulations. Nutricology is the company's consumer brand, and Allergy Research Group is the company's professional (physician's) brand. For more information, call (800) 545-9960 or go to www.nutricology.com.

Thorne Research

Thorne sells its extensive line of high-quality supplements primarily to physicians, but it also accepts orders for most of its products from consumers. For more information, call (208) 263-1337 or go to www.thorne.com.

Natural Food Grocers

I recommend that you eat nutrient-dense fresh and natural foods. Your best bet for finding meat from range- or grass-fed animals and organic fruits and vegetables is a natural foods or specialty grocery store. Always read the fine print on packages to ascertain ingredients.

Trader Joe's

Trader Joe's is a chain of high-quality specialty retail grocery stores, with many organic, gluten-free, and wholesome products. For more information and the locations of Trader Joe's stores, go to www.traderjoes.com.

Vitamin Cottage

This Colorado-based, family-owned group of twenty natural food stores has markets in Denver and other cities in Colorado, as well as in Albuquerque and Santa Fe, New Mexico. For more information and the locations of Vitamin Cottage stores, call (877) 986-4600 or go to www.vitamincottage.com.

Whole Foods

Like Wild Oats, the emphasis is on wholesome, natural foods, including free-range meats, organic produce, and a wide variety of other healthful food products. For more information, go to www.wholefoods.com.

Wild Oats

This national chain emphasizes natural and gourmet foods. Wild Oats' meat departments offer free-range meats. Wild Oats was recently purchased by Whole Foods; the fate of individual Wild Oats stores has not been announced at the time of this book's writing, nor has the overall policy as to whether Wild Oats will keep its name. For more information, call (800) 494-WILD or go to www.wildoats.com.

Specialty Foods Products

Bar Harbor Foods

Herring is rich in quality protein and omega-3 fish oils, but this fish is often ignored by health-conscious people. Bar Harbor Foods, a small company in Maine, markets several types of tasty herring and other fish products that are conveniently packed in small cans. The products include All Natural Wild Herring Fillets, All Natural Wild Herring Fillets in Cabernet Wine Sauce, All Natural Hardwood Smoked Atlantic Mackerel, and All Natural Smoked Wild Kippers. For more information, go to www.barharborfoods.com.

Blue Diamond Natural

This company makes some of the best snack crackers you'll find (called Nut-Thins), all free of wheat and gluten products. They include almond, hazelnut, and pecan Nut-Thins, as well as ranch-flavored almond and cheese-flavored almond Nut-Thins. They're sold at most health and natural food stores. For more information, go to www.bluediamond.com.

Garlic Gold

Rinaldo's Organic Garlic Gold products include several tasty garlic-based products. Among them are Garlic Gold Nuggets, which are toasted garlic pieces that can be substituted for bacon bits, as well as garlic-infused olive oil. For more information, call Seven Oaks Ranch, the manufacturer, at (800) 695-7673, or go to www.garlicgold.com.

Greens8000

One serving of this "greens" drink provides the antioxidant power of twenty servings of fruits and vegetables. It also tastes great, which is rare among similar products. You add one scoop to a glass of water, stir, and drink. Greens8000 is sweetened with stevia and other natural sweeteners (such as spearmint) and contains only 49 calories and 5 grams of carbohydrates per serving. If you have celiac disease, be aware that it may contain trace amounts of gluten (a few parts per million, according to the company), owing to a small amount of barley malt. While Greens8000 should not replace fruits and vegetables in your diet, it is a great way to get extra nutrients that are found in fruits, vegetables, and herbs. For more information, go to www.greens8000.com.

Lara Bars

Lara Bars use simple, nutritious ingredients, such as dates and nuts, to create some of the best-tasting energy bars on the market. They're sold at many health food stores and at Trader Joe's. For more information, go to www.larabar.com.

Lotus Foods

Lotus Foods sells a variety of original and tasty rice and rice flour products, including Bhutanese Red Rice and purple Forbidden Rice. The rice flours can be used to dredge fish and chicken, as well as to make gluten-free crepes. For more information, call (510) 525-3137 or go to www.lotusfoods.com to order or to find recipes.

MacNut Oil (Macadamia Nut Oil)

MacNut Oil, made from Australian macadamia nuts, is rich in oleic acid, the same type of fat that makes olive oil so healthy. MacNut Oil has a slight nutty flavor and a higher smoke point than olive oil. For information, call (866) 462-2688 or go to www.macnutoil.com.

Point Reyes Preserves

This small family-owned business sells some of the best marinated foods (although they're called "pickled" instead of "marinated") in small shops in and around Point Reyes, California, and by mail order. The products include Pickled Asparagus, Pickled Artichoke Hearts, Pickled Mushrooms, Pickled Beets, Pickled Garlic, Pickled Brussels Sprouts, Kosher Dill Pickles, Bread and Butter Pickles, and Corn Relish. All of the products are made from family recipes that have been passed down for generations. All of the vegetables are grown locally, and the products contain no artificial additives or preservatives. For information, go to www.pointreyespreserves.com, e-mail jevans@ horizoncable.com, or write Point Reyes Preserves, P.O. Box 1341, Point Reyes Station, CA 94956.

SELECTED REFERENCES

A complete list of more than three hundred references is available at www.stoppprediabetesnow.com.

Introduction

Diabetes Prevention Program Research Group. Reduction in the incidence of type 2 diabetes with lifestyle intervention or metformin. *New England Journal of Medicine*, 2002;346:393–403.

Duncan GE. Prevalence of diabetes and impaired fasting glucose levels among US adolescents. *Archives of Pediatric and Adolescent Medicine*, 2006;160: 523–528.

Hedley AA, Ogden CL, Johnson CL, et al. Prevalence of overweight and obesity among US children, adolescents, and adults, 1999–2002. *JAMA*, 2004; 291:2847–2850.

Hossain P, Kawar B, El Nahas M. Obesity and diabetes in the developing world—a growing challenge. *New England Journal of Medicine*, 2007;356: 213–215.

Mokdad AH, Ford ES, Bowman BA, et al. Diabetes trends in the U.S.: 1990–1998. *Diabetes Care*, 2000;23:1278–1283.

Narayan KM, Boyle JP, Thompson TJ, et al. Lifetime risk for diabetes mellitus in the United States. *JAMA*, 2003;290:1884–1890.

Ogden CL, Carroll MD, Curtin LR, et al. Prevalence of overweight and obesity in the United States, 1999–2004. *JAMA*, 2006;295:1549–1555.

Pereira MA, Kartashov AI, Ebbeling CB, et al. Fast-food habits, weight gain, and insulin resistance (the CARDIA study): 15-year prospective analysis. *Lancet*, 2005;365:36–42.

Vasan RS, Pencina MJ, Cobain M, et al. Estimated risks for developing obesity in the Framingham heart study. *Annals of Internal Medicine*, 2005;143: 473–480.

Villareal DT, Miller BV, Banks M, et al. Effect of lifestyle intervention on metabolic coronary heart disease risk factors in obese older adults. *American Journal of Clinical Nutrition*, 2006;84:1317–1323.

Wang Y, Rimm EB, Stampfer MJ, et al. Comparison of abdominal adiposity and overall obesity in predicting risk of type 2 diabetes among men. *American Journal of Clinical Nutrition*, 2005;81:555–563.

1. The Prediabetes Problem

Augustin LS, Dal Maso L, La Vecchia C, et al. Dietary glycemic index and glycemic load, and breast cancer risk: a case-control study. *Annals of Oncology*, 2001;12:1533–1538.

Cleland SJ, Petrie JR, Ueda S, et al. Insulin as a vascular hormone: implications for the pathophysiology of cardiovascular disease. *Clinical and Experimental Pharmacology and Physiology*, 1998;25:175–184.

De Lorenzo A, Del Gobbo V, Premrov MG, et al. Normal-weight obese syndrome: early inflammation? *American Journal of Clinical Nutrition*, 2007; 85:40–45.

Kempf K, Rose B, Herder C, et al. Inflammation in metabolic syndrome and type 2 diabetes: impact of dietary glucose. *Annals of the New York Academy of Sciences*, 2006;1084:30–48.

Khaw KT, Wareham N, Bingham S, et al. Association of hemoglobin A_{1c} with cardiovascular disease and mortality in adults: the European prospective investigation into cancer in Norfolk. *Annals of Internal Medicine*, 2004; 141:413–420.

Lev-Ran A. Mitogenic factors accelerate later-age diseases: insulin as a paradigm. *Mechanisms of Aging and Development*, 1998;102:95–113.

Liu S, Manson JE, Buring JE, et al. Relation between a diet with a high glycemic load and plasma concentrations of high-sensitivity C-reactive protein in middle-aged women. *American Journal of Clinical Nutrition*, 2002;75: 492–498.

Love-Osborne K, Butler N, Gao DX, et al. Elevated fasting triglycerides predict impaired glucose tolerance in adolescents at risk for type 2 diabetes. *Pediatric Diabetes*, 2006;7:205–210.

Razay G, Vreugdenhil A, Wilcock G. The metabolic syndrome and Alzheimer disease. *Archives of Neurology*, 2007;64:93–96.

Selvin E, Marinopoulis S, Berkenblit G, et al. Meta-analysis: glycosylated hemoglobin and cardiovascular disease in diabetes mellitus. *Annals of Internal Medicine*, 2004;141:421–431.

Tirosh A, Shai I, Tekes-Manova D, et al. Normal fasting plasma glucose levels and type 2 diabetes in young men. *New England Journal of Medicine*, 2005;353:1454–1462.

Zavaroni I, Bonini L, Gasparini P, et al. Hyperinsulinemia in a normal population as a predictor of non-insulin-dependent diabetes mellitus, hypertension, and coronary heart disease: the Barilla factory revisited. *Metabolism*, 1999;48:989–994.

2. Food Isn't What It Used to Be

Malik VS, Schulze MB, Hu FB. Intake of sugar-sweetened beverages and weight gain: a systematic review. *American Journal of Clinical Nutrition*, 2006;84:274–288.

Plotnick GD, Corretti MC, Vogel RA. Effect of antioxidant vitamins on the transient impairment of endothelium-dependent brachial artery vasoactivity following a single high-fat meal. *JAMA*, 1997;278:1682–1686.

Yanovski JA, Yanovski SZ, Sovik KN, et al. A prospective study of holiday weight gain. *New England Journal of Medicine*, 2000;342:861–867.

3. Dangers That Lurk beyond Calories and Carbs

Anderson C, Horne JA. A high sugar content, low caffeine drink does not alleviate sleepiness but may worsen it. *Human Psychopharmacology*, 2006;21: 299–303.

Brownlee C. Food fix: neurobiology highlights similarities between obesity and drug addiction. *Science News*, 2005;168:155–156.

Cooney CA, Dave AA, Wolff GL. Maternal methyl supplements in mice affect epigenetic variation and DNA methylation of offspring. *Journal of Nutrition*, 2002;132:2392S–2400S.

Costa AG, Bressan J, Sabarense CM. Trans fatty acids: foods and effects on health. *Archivos Latinoamericanos de Nutrición*, 2006 Mar;56(1):12–21.

Elliott SS, Keim NL, Stern JS, et al. Fructose, weight gain, and the insulin resistance syndrome. *American Journal of Clinical Nutrition*, 2002;76:911–922.

Farshchi HR, Taylor MA, Macdonald IA. Deleterious effects of omitting breakfast on insulin sensitivity and fasting lipid profiles in healthy lean women. *American Journal of Clinical Nutrition*, 2005;81:388–396.

Feinman RD, Fine EJ. "A calorie is a calorie" violates the second law of thermodynamics. *Nutrition Journal*, 2004;3:9–13.

Hill EG, Johnson SB, Lawson LD, et al. Perturbation of the metabolism of essential fatty acids by dietary partially hydrogenated vegetable oil. *Proceedings of the National Academy of Sciences*, 1982;79:953–957.

Johnston CS. Strategies for healthy weight loss: from vitamin C to the glycemic response. *Journal of the American College of Nutrition*, 2005;24:158–165.

Liljeberg HGM, Akerberg AKE, Bjorck IME. Effect of the glycemic index and content of indigestible carbohydrates of cereal-based breakfast meals on glucose tolerance at lunch in healthy subjects. *American Journal of Clinical Nutrition*, 1999;69:647–655.

Ludwig DS. The Glycemic Index. Physiological mechanisms relating to obesity, diabetes, and cardiovascular disease. *JAMA*, 2002;287:2414–2423.

Mazaffarian D, Katan MB, Ascherio A, et al. Trans fatty acids and cardiovascular disease. *New England Journal of Medicine*, 2006;354:1601–1613.

Pittas AG, Das SK, Hajduk CL, et al. A low-glycemic load diet facilitates greater weight loss in overweight adults with high insulin secretion but not in overweight adults with low insulin secretion in the CALERIE trial. *Diabetes Care*, 2005;28:2939–2941.

Sundram K, Karupaiah T, Hayes KC. Stearic acid-rich interesterified fat and trans-rich fat raise the LDL/HDL ratio and plasma glucose relative to palm olein in humans. *Nutrition & Metabolism*, 2007;4:3.

Teng RZW, Szeto CC, Chan MHM, et al. Risk factors of vitamin B12 deficiency in patients receiving metformin. *Archives of Internal Medicine*, 2006; 166:1975–1979.

Vander Wal JS, Marth JM, Khosla P, et al. Short-term effect of eggs on satiety in overweight and obese subjects. *Journal of the American College of Nutrition*, 2005;24:510–515.

4. Easy Ways to Curb Your Appetite

Borzoel S, Neovius M, Barkeling B, et al. A comparison of effects of fish and beef protein on satiety in normal weight men. *European Journal of Clinical Nutrition*, 2006;60:897–902.

Fujioka K, Greenway F, Sheard J, et al. The effects of grapefruit on weight and insulin resistance: relationship to the metabolic syndrome. *Journal of Medicinal Food*, 2006;9:49–54.

Gannon MC, Nuttall FQ. Effect of a high-protein, low-carbohydrate diet on blood glucose control in people with type 2 diabetes. *Diabetes*, 2004;53: 2375–2382.

Halton TL, Willett WC, Liu S, et al. Low-carbohydrate-diet score and the risk of coronary heart disease in women. *New England Journal of Medicine*, 2006;355:1991–2002.

Hodge AM, English DR, O'Dea K, et al. Glycemic index and dietary fiber and the risk of type 2 diabetes. *Diabetes Care*, 2004;27:2701–2706.

Johnston CS, Kim CM, Buller AJ. Vinegar improves insulin sensitivity to a high-carbohydrate meal in subjects with insulin resistance or type 2 diabetes. *Diabetes Care*, 2004;27:281–282.

Layman DK, Baum JI. Dietary protein impact on glycemic control during weight loss. *Journal of Nutrition*, 2004;134:968S–973S.

Layman DK, Evans E, Baum JI, et al. Dietary protein and exercise have additive effects on body composition during weight loss in adult women. *Journal of Nutrition*, 2005;135:1903–1910.

Manninen AH. Very-low-carbohydrate diets and preservation of muscle mass. *Nutrition & Metabolism*, 2006;3:9–12.

5. Improve Your Relationship with Food

David DR, Epp MD, Riordan HD. Changes in USDA Food Composition Data for 43 Garden Crops, 1950 to 1999. *Journal of the American College of Nutrition*, 2004;23:669–682.

Delarue J, DeFoll C, Corporeau C, et al. N-3 long chain polyunsaturated fatty acids: a nutritional tool to prevent insulin resistance associated to type 2 diabetes and obesity? *Reproduction, Nutrition, Development*, 2004;44:289–299.

Jenkins DJ, Kendal CW, Josse AR, et al. Almonds decrease postprandial glycemia, insulinemia, and oxidative damage in healthy individuals. *Journal of Nutrition*, 2006;136:2987–2992.

Seiquer I, Diaz-Alguacil J, Delgado-Andrade C, et al. Diets rich in Maillard reaction products affect protein digestibility in adolescent males aged 11–14 y. *American Journal of Clinical Nutrition*, 2006;83:1082–1088.

Wansink B, Chandon P. Meal size, not body size, explains errors in estimating the calorie contents of meals. *Annals of Internal Medicine*, 2006;145: 326–332.

6. Figure Out What Food Labels Really Mean

Bell RR, Spencer MJ, Sherriff JL. Voluntary exercise and monounsaturated canola oil reduce fat gain in mice fed diets high in fat. *Journal of Nutrition*, 1997;127:2006–2010.

Rothman RL, Housam R, Weiss H, et al. Patient understanding of food labels: the role of literacy and numeracy. *American Journal of Preventive Medicine*, 2006;31:391–398.

Salmeron J, Hu FB, Manson JE, et al. Dietary fat intake and risk of type 2 diabetes in men. *American Journal of Clinical Nutrition*, 2001;73:1019–1026.

9. Navigate Restaurants and Menus

DeCastro JM. Family and friends produce greater social facilitation of food-intake than other companions. *Physiology and Behavior*, 1994;56:445–455.

DeCastro JM. Eating behavior: lessons from the real world of humans. *Ingestive Behavior and Obesity*, 2000;16:800–813.

Duffey KJ, Gordon-Larsen P, Jacobs DR, et al. Differential associations of fast food and restaurant food consumption with 3-y change in body mass index: the coronary artery risk development in young adults study. *American Journal of Clinical Nutrition*, 2007;85:201–208.

10. The Best Supplements for Improving Blood Sugar

Anderson RA, Chen N, Bryden NA, et al. Elevated intakes of supplemental chromium improve glucose and insulin variables in individuals with type 2 diabetes. *Diabetes*, 1997;46:1786–1791.

Cigolini M, Iagulli MP, Miconi V, et al. Serum 25-hydroxyvitamin D3 concentrations and prevalence of cardiovascular disease among type 2 diabetic patients. *Diabetes Care*, 2006;29:722–724.

Johnston CS, Corte C, Swan PD. Marginal vitamin C status is associated with reduced fat oxidation during submaximal exercise in young adults. *Nutrition & Metabolism*, 2006;3:35.

Kilic-Okman T, Kucuk M. N-acetylcysteine treatment for polycystic ovary syndrome. *International Journal of Gynecology & Obstetrics*, 2004;85:296–297.

Kim HK, Della-Fera M, Baile CA. Docosahexaenoic acid inhibits adipocyte differentiation and induces apoptosis in 3T3-L1 preadipocytes. *Journal of Nutrition*, 2006;136:2965–2969.

Kim MS, Park JY, Namkoong C, et al. Anti-obesity effects of a-lipoic acid mediated by suppression of hypothalamic AMP-activated protein kinase. *Nature Medicine*, 2004;10:727–733.

Koopman R, Verdijk L, Manders RJ, et al. Co-ingestion of protein and leucine stimulates muscle protein synthesis rates to the same extent in young and elderly lean men. *American Journal of Clinical Nutrition*, 2006;84:623–632.

Mehdi MZ, Pandey SK, Theberge JF, et al. Insulin signal mimicry as a mechanism for the insulin-like effects of vanadium. *Cell Biochemistry and Biophysics*, 2006;44:73–81.

Packer L, Kraemer K, Rimbach G. Molecular aspects of lipoic acid in the prevention of diabetes complications. *Nutrition*, 2001;17:888–895.

Rennie MJ. A role for leucine in rejuvenating the anabolic effects of food in old rats. *Journal of Physiology*, 2005;569:357.

Song Y, He K, Levitan EB, et al. Effects of oral magnesium supplementation on glycaemic control in type 2 diabetes: a meta-analysis of randomized double-blind controlled trials. *Diabetic Medicine*, 2006;23:1050–1056.

Velussi M, Cernigoi AM, De Monte AD, et al. Long-term (12 months) treatment with an antioxidant drug (silymarin) is effective on hyperinsulinemia, exogenous insulin need and malondialdehyde levels in cirrhotic diabetic patients. *Journal of Hepatology*, 1997;26:871–879.

Vuksan V, Sievenpiper JL, Koo VYY, et al. American ginseng (panax quinquefolius L) reduces postprandial glycemia in nondiabetic subjects and subjects with type 2 diabetes mellitus. *Archives of Internal Medicine*, 2000;160:1009–1013.

11. Overcome Related Health Problems

Ahlberg AC, Ljung T, Rosmond R, et al. Depression and anxiety symptoms in relation to anthropometry and metabolism in men. *Psychiatry Research*, 2002;112:101–110.

Alvarez-Blasco F, Botella-Carretero JI, San Millan JL, et al. Prevalence and characteristics of polycystic ovary syndrome in overweight and obese women. *Archives of Internal Medicine*, 2006;166:2081–2086.

Bacon CG, Mittleman MA, Kawachi I, et al. A prospective study of risk factors for erectile dysfunction. *Journal of Urology*, 2006;176:217–221.

Burdakov D, Lensen LT, Alexopoulos H, et al. Tandem-pore K+ channels mediate inhibition of orexin neurons by glucose. *Neuron*, 2006;50:711–722.

Cavallini G, Caracciolo S, Vitali G, et al. Carnitine versus androgen administration in the treatment of sexual dysfunction, depressed mood, and fatigue associated with male aging. *Urology*, 2004;63:641–646.

Chandola T, Brunner E, Marmot M. Chronic stress at work and the metabolic syndrome: prospective study. *British Medical Journal*, 2006;332:521–525.

Demirbag R, Yilmaz R, Gur M, et al. DNA damage in metabolic syndrome and its association with antioxidative and oxidative measurements. *International Journal of Clinical Practice*, 2006;60:1187–1193.

Gottlieb DJ, Punjabi NM, Newman AB, et al. Association of sleep time with diabetes mellitus and impaired glucose tolerance. *Archives of Internal Medicine*, 2005;165:863–868.

Griffin MD, Sanders TAB, Davies IG, et al. Effects of altering the ratio of dietary n-6 to n-3 fatty acids on insulin sensitivity, lipoprotein size, and postprandial lipemia in men and postmenopausal women aged 45–70 y: the OPTILIP study. *American Journal of Clinical Nutrition*, 2006;84:1290–1298.

Henry EB, Carswell A, Wirz A, et al. Proton pump inhibitors reduce the bioavailability of dietary vitamin C. *Alimentary Pharmacology & Therapeutics*, 2005;22:539–545.

Inoue M, Iwasaki M, Otani T, et al. Diabetes mellitus and the risk of cancer. *Archives of Internal Medicine*, 2006;166:1871–1877.

Kaplan SA, Meehan AG, Shah A. The age related decrease in testosterone is significantly exacerbated in obese men with the metabolic syndrome. What are the implications for the relatively high incidence of erectile dysfunction observed in these men? *Journal of Urology*, 2006;176:1524–1527.

Kilic-Okman T, Kucuk M. N-acetylcysteine treatment for polycystic ovary syndrome. *International Journal of Gynecology & Obstetrics*, 2004;85:296–297.

Knutson KL, Ryden AM, Mander BA, et al. Role of sleep duration and quality in the risk and severity of type 2 diabetes mellitus. *Archives of Internal Medicine*, 2006;166:1768–1774.

McKay D. Nutrients and botanicals for erectile dysfunction: examining the evidence. *Alternative Medicine Review*, 2004;9:4–16.

McVeigh KH, Mostashari F, Thorpe LE. Serious psychological distress among persons with diabetes—New York City, 2003. *Morbidity and Mortality Weekly Report*, November 26, 2004;53;1089–1092.

Mills DE, Prkachin KM, Harvey KA, et al. Dietary fatty acid supplementation alters stress reactivity and performance in man. *Journal of Human Hypertension*, 1989;3:111–116.

Naegele B, Launois SH, Mazza S, et al. Which memory processes are affected in patients with obstructive sleep apnea? An evaluation of 3 types of memory. *Sleep*, 2006;29:533–544.

Tarkun I, Arsian BC, Canturk Z, et al. Endothelial dysfunction in young women with polycystic ovary syndrome: relationship with insulin resistance and low-grade chronic inflammation. *Journal of Clinical Endocrinology and Metabolism*, 2004;89:5592–5596.

Travison TG, Araujo AB, Kupelian V, et al. The relative contributions of aging, health, and lifestyle factors to serum testosterone decline in men. *Journal of Endocrinology and Metabolism*, 2006:epub ahead of print.

Vorona RD, Winn MP, Babineau TW, et al. Overweight and obese patients in a primary care population report less sleep than patients with a normal body mass index. *Archives of Internal Medicine*, 2005;165:25–30.

Yang YX, Lewis JD, Epstein S, et al. Long-term proton pump inhibitor therapy and risk of hip fracture. *JAMA*, 2006;292:2947–2953.

12. Get More Active and Actually Enjoy It

Dunstan DW, Vulikh E, Owen N, et al. Community center–based resistance training for the maintenance of glycemic control in adults with type 2 diabetes. *Diabetes Care*, 2006;29:2586–2591.

Franco OH, de Laet C, Peeters A, et al. Effects of physical activity on life expectancy with cardiovascular disease. *Archives of Internal Medicine*, 2005;165:2355–2360.

Giannopoulou I, Ploutz-Snyder LL. Exercise is required for visceral fat loss in postmenopausal women with type 2 diabetes. *Journal of Clinical Endocrinology and Metabolism*, 2005;90:1511–1518.

Ibanez J, Izquierdo M, Arguelles I, et al. Twice-weekly progressive resistance training decreases abdominal fat and improves insulin sensitivity in older men with type 2 diabetes. *Diabetes Care*, 2005;28:662–667.

Layman DK, Evans E, Baum JI, et al. Dietary protein and exercise have additive effects on body composition during weight loss in adult women. *Journal of Nutrition*, 2005;135:1903–1910.

Weiss EP, Racette SB, Willareal DT, et al. Improvements in glucose tolerance and insulin action induced by increasing energy expenditure or decreasing energy intake: a randomized controlled trial. *American Journal of Clinical Nutrition*, 2006;84:1033–1042.

You T, Murphy KM, Lyles MF, et al. Addition of aerobic exercise to dietary weight loss preferentially reduces abdominal adipocyte size. *International Journal of Obesity*, 2006;30:1211–1216.

INDEX